The
Healthy Heart
Walking Book

The Healthy Heart Walking Book

THE AMERICAN HEART ASSOCIATION

MACMILLAN • USA

This book is not intended as a substitute for medical advice of physicians. The reader should regularly consult a physician in matters relating to his or her health and particularly in respect of any symptoms which might require diagnosis or medical attention.

MACMILLAN
A Simon & Schuster Macmillan Company
1633 Broadway
New York, NY 10019–6785

MACMILLAN is a registered trademark of Macmillan, Inc.

Library of Congress Cataloging-in-Publication Data
The healthy heart walking book / American Heart Association.
        p. cm.
    Includes index.
    ISBN 0-02-860447-4
    1. Fitness walking.   2. Walking—Health aspects.   I. American
Heart Association.
RA781.65.H43   1995   95-22491
613.7'176—dc20   CIP

Produced by March Tenth, Inc.
Designed by Stanley S. Drate/Folio Graphics Co., Inc.

10   9   8   7   6   5   4   3   2   1

Printed in the United States of America

CONTENTS

～

ACKNOWLEDGMENTS   vii

INTRODUCTION   ix

CHAPTER 1   Why Exercise?   1

CHAPTER 2   Why Choose Walking?   9

CHAPTER 3   Before You Start   25

CHAPTER 4   F.I.T.T. for Life   36

CHAPTER 5   On Your Mark!   49

CHAPTER 6   Get Set!   57

CHAPTER 7   Let's Go for a Walk!   66

CHAPTER 8   Staying Motivated   86

CHAPTER 9   Advanced Walking   97

CHAPTER 10   Balancing Your Fitness Program   102

CHAPTER 11   Eating for Health and Fitness   110

CHAPTER 12   Injuries Are a Pain   117

CHAPTER 13   Special Cases   122

CHAPTER 14   How to Track Down Walking
              Opportunities   128

APPENDIX I: The Walking Diary   141

APPENDIX II: Scoring the One-Mile Fitness Test   169

APPENDIX III: Personal Data Record   171

APPENDIX IV: Walking Milestones   173

APPENDIX V: American Heart Association Affiliates   175

INDEX   177

ACKNOWLEDGMENTS

The real secret of success is enthusiasm.
—WALTER CHRYSLER

If ever a team of experts had fun with a project, this is it. The staff at the American Heart Association and the Cooper Institute for Aerobics Research are passionate about walking. And we have tried to convey our love in these pages.

Why? Because we've seen it help bring heart attack patients back to a fully active life. We've seen it keep people active and vigorous well into their eighties, nineties, and beyond. And we all know from experience how great it feels to have a healthy heart. We wrote this book because that's our wish for you.

The first truckload of thanks goes to the staff of the Cooper Institute for Aerobics Research, a non-profit preventive medicine research and education center in Dallas, Texas. Project directors Ruth Ann Carpenter, M.S., R.D., and Brenda S. Mitchell, Ph.D., wrote much of the text. Sara Kelling, M.P.H., R.D., also made major contributions.

Meanwhile, thanks go to Sam Inman, Debra Ebel, Barbara Jenkins, and Ann Yanosky, of the American Heart Association's Corporate Relations staff, for facilitating the collaboration between the AHA and Macmillan.

AHA Consumer Publications Consultant Peter Landesman gathered the team of experts, writers, and editors. Senior Editor Jane Ruehl managed the editorial process of transforming the idea into the book. Writer Pat Naegele crafted the words of the experts into user-friendly text.

On hand to double-check scientific accuracy was Science Consultant Terry Bazzarre, Ph.D., FACSM. And the almost continual science review was coordinated by Sherry Read.

These talented people put their hearts and souls and soles into this project. They researched, wrote, worked, and (naturally) walked about a million miles in the process. They hope that this book will inspire you.

INTRODUCTION

﹏

Feeling lethargic? Your life's on hold . . . energy's drained. . . .

Well, you've come to the right place. The American Heart Association knows that walking is more than just a way to keep your heart healthy. It's a whole new way of life. It helps you meet people. It boosts your energy. And, frankly, it's *fun!*

For more than seventy years, the AHA has been on your side against America's number one killer, heart disease. Our mission is to reduce disability and death from cardiovascular diseases and stroke. This book is part of that mission. We hope it will lure you into walking as a way of life. And we mean *life.*

Move It Or Lose It

A few years ago, scientific research confirmed that physical inactivity is a major risk factor for heart disease. We now know that people who are sedentary have a much greater chance of developing heart disease—and dying from it. At the same time, we learned that you don't have to run a marathon every day to protect your heart. Moderate exercise—like regular walking—will do it.

On these pages, we've given you all the information and tools you need to make walking a lifetime habit. You'll learn:

☐ What walking can do for you
☐ Your current fitness level
☐ How to start slow and pick up your pace
☐ The best places to walk
☐ How to find good walking shoes
☐ What to eat for optimum health and fitness
☐ How to stay motivated
☐ How to walk if you have a health condition
☐ How to put more walking into your life

And you'll find your own twelve-week walking diary built right into the book. You can personalize it by customizing it to your needs. No other walking book on the market contains a complete walking log and diary.

The Healthy Heart Walking Book is like the AHA itself: It's ready to help anyone, anytime, any place. It's not just for couch potatoes. It's not just for jocks. The truth is, no matter what your age or fitness level, this book can help you. It carries you step by step through a walking program that's custom made for you based on your current fitness level. What if you don't like the traditional exercise approach? No problem. We show you how to build walking into your daily routine. That way, you can get heart-protecting exercise that seems like a natural part of your day, not a formal "program." We call it the "lifestyle" approach to walking.

To Life!

At the American Heart Association, we hope this book will help you take control of your life and health. Over the years, we've learned that some people simply want to put more years into their lives and more life into their years. They're the ones who are doing something about it. We expect to see you out there with them.

Here's to life!

CHAPTER

1

Why Exercise?

To Work Out Or Not to Work Out . . .

That *is* the question. Is it healthier to exercise than to be a couch potato? Most of us know the answer. Of course it is! But *knowing* and *doing* are two different things. Surveys show that 24 percent of American adults are total sofa spuds. They're not active at all. On the other hand, most adults (54 percent) get *some* exercise. They just don't do it regularly or intensely enough to protect their heart. Only 22 percent of American adults get enough leisure time exercise to net any health benefits.

So why don't more people exercise? Maybe it's because they don't know just how much regular exercise can help them. The fact is that regular physical activity can do a whole lot more than most people ever imagine. It can help:

- ☐ reduce your risk of heart disease
- ☐ keep your weight under control
- ☐ improve your blood cholesterol levels
- ☐ prevent and manage high blood pressure
- ☐ prevent bone loss
- ☐ boost your energy level
- ☐ manage tension
- ☐ improve your self-image
- ☐ counter anxiety and depression

☐ increase your muscle strength, giving you a greater capacity for other physical activities

You may have more reasons for wanting to be active. List them below. Feel free to add to the list as you think of more reasons.

Why I Want To Be More Active

In the space below, list your reasons for wanting to lead a physically active lifestyle.

_____

_____

_____

_____

_____

_____

WHAT'S HOLDING YOU BACK?

Too many people have excuses for not exercising. These excuses can become barriers to leading an active, enjoyable life. If any of these common barriers apply to you, read on.

- *I don't have the time.*

Let's face it, we're all busy. Fortunately, all it takes to get the health benefits you need is 30 minutes or more of moderate exercise on most days of the week. And you don't have to do it all at once. For example, take the stairs at work instead of the elevator. Park your car farther away from the office and walk in. Take your dog for a daily walk. Three 10-minute exercise sessions add up to the 30 minutes you need!

- *I don't have the energy. I always feel tired.*

We all feel tired some of the time. The fact is, being inactive and physically unfit can actually make you feel tired. Ironically, when people start exercising, they report feeling more energetic than ever before. Stress and lack of physical activity can zap your energy. Regular physical activity can help relieve stress—and boost your energy level.

- *I've never liked to exercise.*

Exercise is *not* medieval torture. In fact, it's supposed to be *fun*—that's one reason why people do it. Unfortunately, some people associate exercise with negative images. They think of basic training in the military or grueling "no pain, no gain" gym classes. Some may remember the agony of not being chosen for gym-class teams. If that sounds familiar to you, take a breather, and change the picture in your head. Studies show that you don't have to be a jock to benefit from regular exercise. Many of the things you already enjoy—like walking or gardening—can improve your health. The trick is to do them on most days. Making exercise fun is vitally important. Choose something you like to do, stick with it, and *have fun.*

- *It costs too much.*

You don't have to spend hundreds of dollars on health club memberships and home fitness equipment. You can be physically active without expensive equipment. Just find ways to build activity into your normal day. For a walking program, all you need is a good pair of walking shoes—and the willingness to move out of your comfort zone.

- *I'm too old.*

That's just a myth. In fact, more and more seniors are proving that every day. It's true that some people become less physically active as they get older. But remember: The older you are, the more you need regular exercise. It helps prevent bone loss and reduces the risk of dozens of diseases. It also improves your capacity for basic living, making it easier to carry grocery bags, get up from a chair, and take care of household chores. Age is no longer an excuse. If you can walk to the telephone, you can walk around the block. Being physically active is a real key in maintaining your quality of life.

- *I have other health problems.*

If that's the case, please check with your doctor before beginning any exercise program. But remember this: Active people with high blood pressure, high blood cholesterol, diabetes, or other chronic diseases are less likely to die prematurely than inactive people with these conditions.

- *I don't want to get injured or have a heart attack.*

  We're with you on this one! And we have good news on both fronts.

  First, there are ways you can help prevent injuries. Just start slowly and gradually increase your physical activity level. Be sure to wear comfortable clothing and shoes that fit. We'll take you through all these steps in Chapter 6. Many activities, such as walking and running, don't require any special skills. Others, such as biking and roller-blading, require special equipment and a little skill. Find the activity you feel most comfortable with, and take it slow.

  Second, having a heart attack during exercise is extremely rare. When it does happen, it usually involves a person who already has a heart condition. The fact is that being physically active actually *reduces* your risk of a sudden, fatal heart attack. It can also help reduce your risk of a second heart attack. If you have particular concerns, discuss them with your doctor. Just start with a slow and easy exercise plan, and be sure to listen to your body.

What Are Your Activity Barriers?

Check off the exercise barriers that apply to you. You may wish to add others not listed here.

____ I don't have the time	____ I'm afraid of injury
____ I don't have the energy	____ I have other health concerns
____ I don't like to exercise	_____
____ I don't have the money	_____
____ I'm too old	_____
____ I'm afraid of the risk of a heart attack	_____

JUST DO IT

Do you want to know a good way to get started on an exercise program? Choose an activity you enjoy. *Any* activity. Really, it's that simple. The important thing is to do *something*. Think of your life as being full of choices. Your choices can be positive or negative, or you can choose the procrastinator's option, which is no choice. But if you want to enjoy life, then consider these positive approaches to a healthy, happy, active lifestyle.

Research clearly shows that doing *any* physical activity is better than doing nothing. Even low-intensity activities, like gardening, housework, and leisure walking, can provide long-term benefits, including lowering your risk of heart disease. Once you start being more physically active, you'll be surprised at how good you feel. And you'll get other rewards from being active (see the list on pages 17–18). For even more benefits, simply build up to moderate and then to more vigorous activities. Try to do these activities for 30 minutes or longer at least four days a week.

Most of the barriers that keep you from exercising can be removed or overcome. That's what this book is all about. It will show you how to build physical activity into your everyday life. It will also show you how to start a healthy walking program. But before we focus on walking, let's look at the three main types of physical activity and why each is important to your good health.

The Major Types of Physical Activity

There are three major types of physical activity, and they each help you in a different way. *Aerobic exercises,* such as walking, jogging, and swimming, can improve your heart and lung capacity. These are exercises that increase cardiovascular fitness. *Strength training exercises,* such as weightlifting, can strengthen and tone the major muscles in your legs, arms, back, and abdomen. *Stretching activities,* such as yoga or gymnastics, can help your muscles and joints stay flexible. All three types of physical activities are important for your overall fitness, good health, and function. Since walking is an aerobic activity, let's take a closer look at cardiovascular fitness. Strength training and stretching activities are discussed in greater detail on pages 103–106.

CARDIOVASCULAR FITNESS: A WORKOUT FOR YOUR HEART

Regular aerobic exercise gives your heart and lungs a workout. This strengthens your heart muscle, your lungs, and your entire cardiovascular system. And it will reduce your risk of heart disease.

Aerobic activities are those that cause your heart to beat faster and your breathing to be heavier. They use the large muscle groups of your legs, back, and arms in a continuous and rhythmic manner. As you move, your body needs more oxygen (hence the term *aerobic*) to produce the energy needed to move these muscles. This activity challenges your heart, lungs, and blood vessels to work harder and get oxygen and blood to those hard-working muscles.

Like any other muscle in your body, your heart adapts to this increased workload over time by becoming stronger. As it gets stronger your heart becomes more efficient and pumps more blood with each beat.

And here's a bonus: Aerobic activity can reduce blood pressure. Research has shown that some people who use medicine to control their blood pressure may be able to reduce the dosage or even eliminate it when they exercise regularly. Also, moderate-to-vigorous aerobic exercise can increase your HDL-cholesterol; that's high density lipoprotein, the so-called "good" cholesterol in your blood. HDL-cholesterol has been linked to a lower risk of heart disease.

Exercise can also help you lose weight and feel more energized. Finally, regular exercise can reduce your risk of other chronic health problems such as diabetes and osteoporosis.

There are many different types of aerobic activities. The key is to find one (or more!) that you enjoy. Then be sure to exercise at a level that is right for you, whether it's anything from a low intensity to a very vigorous workout. The important thing is to find a level that is right for you and stick with it. As you become more fit, you may want to add more vigorous activities to your workout. We'll talk about that later.

VIGOROUS AEROBIC ACTIVITIES

To improve your heart and lungs, aerobic activity must be brisk, sustained, and regular. Vigorous aerobic activities, such as the ones listed below, are especially helpful when you do them regularly. The American Heart Association recommends that you do at least 30 minutes of aerobic activity three or four times a week. This activity should be at more than 50 percent of your exercise capacity. (We'll get to this on page 42 when we discuss your target heart rate zone.) As a bonus, vigorous aerobic activities burn more calories than less vigorous ones.

VIGOROUS AEROBIC ACTIVITIES

- Aerobic Dancing
- Bicycling
- Cross-country Skiing
- Hiking
- Ice Hockey
- Jogging and Running
- Jumping Rope
- Rowing
- Skating
- Stair-climbing
- Stationary Cycling
- Swimming
- Walking Briskly

MODERATE AEROBIC ACTIVITIES

Moderate activities are excellent choices for a physical activity program. When you exercise moderately for 30 minutes or longer three or four times a week you will also condition your heart and lungs. And you'll find you can sustain moderate activities much longer than vigorous ones. In fact, it's possible that you'll burn more calories doing a longer routine of moderate exercise than a shorter one of vigorous exercise. Also, there's less risk of injury. For some people, a program of moderate exercise is the key.

MODERATE AEROBIC ACTIVITIES

- Calisthenics
- Tennis (singles)
- Dancing
- Field Hockey
- Volleyball
- Walking Moderately

LOW-INTENSITY ACTIVITIES

Low-intensity or short-duration activities are not aerobic. That's because you're not involving your heart and lungs to any great extent. These activities probably won't condition your heart and lungs unless you do them every day or unless you have been extremely sedentary.

Even so, these activities can help you improve muscle tone and coordination, relieve tension, and burn some calories. They're a good place to start if you haven't been active for a long time. Gradually work your way up to more vigorous activities as your cardiovascular system gets stronger. This system allows your body to adapt to each new level of activity. You may want to move from walking at an easy pace to walking at a brisk pace. Or you may want to move from a leisurely swim to a faster swim. The important thing is to stay active and enjoy yourself.

LOW-INTENSITY ACTIVITIES
(Not Vigorous or Sustained)

- Badminton
- Baseball
- Bowling
- Croquet
- Football
- Light Gardening
- Golf (on foot or by cart)

- Housework (vacuuming, mowing the yard)
- Ping-Pong
- Shuffleboard
- Social Dancing
- Softball
- Walking Leisurely

WALK AWAY WITH A HEALTHY HEART

You'll notice that we've included walking in each type of aerobic activity. In many ways, walking is an ideal exercise because you can do it at any intensity level. That's one of the reasons we wrote this book. In Chapter 4, we'll help you find the walking plan that's right for you.

Why Choose Walking?

Choose An Activity, Any Activity

Swimming, cycling, jogging, skiing, aerobic dancing, or any of dozens of other activities can help your heart. They all cause you to feel warm, perspire, and breathe heavily without being out of breath and without feeling any burning sensation in your muscles. All these exercises and, in fact, any physical activity that gets your heart pumping is better than doing nothing at all. Whether it's a structured exercise program or just part of your daily routine, all exercise adds up to a healthier heart. The tough thing is choosing the cardiovascular exercise that is best for you. Try not to rely too much on one special activity, but develop a repertoire of several that you can enjoy. That way you'll never view exercise as boring and routine. A good way to start is to get the full story on different activities that appeal to you. Consider the cost of getting started, when and where you can do it, and how challenging it will be. For many people, walking is the natural choice. It is a great foundation activity that you can do at home, at work, or when you're traveling. In this chapter, we'll compare walking to other types of exercise.

The Heart and Sole of Walking

Walking offers so many benefits that it's easy to see why it is one of the most popular forms of exercise in America today. Remember, walking is neither better nor worse than other exercises. But it does have several unique features to recommend it, especially if you're getting up off that couch for the first time.

AMERICA'S FAVORITE EXERCISE

All things considered, walking compares favorably with other cardiovascular fitness activities. It's inexpensive, easy, and convenient. Plus, you're more likely to *keep* walking for exercise throughout your lifetime. In fact, walking boasts the highest adherence rate and lowest dropout rate of any physical activity. It's clearly the exercise of choice for most adults.

WALKING CHALLENGES YOUR HEART, NOT YOUR BODY

Walking is a low-impact, weight-bearing exercise. While it gives your heart and blood vessels a workout, it exerts only one-fifth the force of jogging on your bones and joints. Yet it also offers the benefits of weight-bearing exercise. Weight-bearing exercise, such as weightlifting or running, can help slow down the bone loss that occurs with normal aging and the serious bone-loss condition known as osteoporosis.

By contrast, jogging, stair-climbing, racquet sports, and vigorous aerobic dance are high-impact, weight-bearing activities. While they are excellent workouts for your heart, they require greater skill and are hard on your joints. These may not be recommended if you've had a previous injury, chronic arthritis, or other joint problems.

LITTLE COST, BIG BENEFITS

You can start walking today without spending big bucks. That's because you don't need special equipment other than a comfortable pair of walking shoes. Other types of exercise often require major investments in equipment.

Cardiovascular exercise equipment such as treadmills, rowing machines, stair-climbing machines, stationary cycles, and ski machines are great for home use. Such equipment, however, is likely to cost several hundred dollars. If you buy your own exercise equipment, maintenance and repairs are another consideration. Can you do the repairs yourself? If not, how will you handle repairs? Can you take the item to a shop for repairs, or must you have someone come to your home? Not having the equipment readily available because of breakdowns could cost you more than time and money. It could also interrupt your routine and cause you to stop exercising.

What do you do if you get tired of the equipment or no longer want it? We all know someone who has a stationary cycle or rowing machine gathering dust in the basement, garage, or attic. Many people purchase these items on a whim. Then they may discover that they don't really like doing that form of exercise. So, it may be best to wait until you're sure you'll stick with an exercise before making major investments in equipment.

Another option is to go to a recreation center, health club, or fitness center. Most of these facilities charge a fee, which is sometimes very high. And you may have to wait in line to use the equipment. If swimming is your exercise of choice, finding a pool is often a problem.

If you enjoy sports, remember they often require an investment in equipment and accessories, although they generally are not as expensive as cardiovascular exercise machines. You'll need a racquet and balls to play tennis, racquetball, and squash. To bike, you'll need a bicycle, helmet, and other accessories.

For walking, all you need is a good pair of walking shoes. Just put them on and go. Depending on the weather, you may not even have to change clothes. And it's easy to carry a pair of walking shoes with you. You can now find several brands of walking shoes styled for dress or business attire that are extremely comfortable.

LOCATION, LOCATION, LOCATION

Finding a safe and convenient place to exercise is sometimes difficult. Here again, walking has the edge, because you can walk almost anywhere, including areas that are not suitable for jogging, running, or cycling, almost any time you want. Almost all walkers have a favorite place to walk.

FAVORITE WALKING TIMES AND PLACES

Here are a few all-time favorites. Add new ideas as you discover them.

☐ School or college tracks
☐ Shopping malls

☐ Neighborhood sidewalks
☐ Park trails
☐ Parking lots
☐ Airline terminals (while waiting for a plane)
☐ Special events (walk-a-thon, fun run)
☐ Hiking trails
☐ Walking tours
☐ Museums
☐ Anywhere you can walk the dog
☐ Walking with a baby/stroller
☐ _____
☐ _____
☐ _____
☐ _____
☐ _____

YOU CAN HAVE IT YOUR WAY

Only walking gives you the opportunity to solo, double up, or go with the gang—as the mood strikes. If you want company, it's easy to carry on a conversation while walking. But you also can use your walking time to think, plan, or just chill out, if that's what you want.

A LOW-RISK WORKOUT

Most exercise is safe for any healthy adult, and walking is especially so. If you have a chronic disease, such as heart disease, high blood pressure, diabetes, asthma, or arthritis, check with your doctor before starting. Chances are he or she will approve a moderate walking program.

The risk of a bone, muscle, or joint injury from walking is remote because it's a low-impact activity. And with walking you're not as likely to feel the muscle soreness common to people who first take up jogging, swimming, cycling, or aerobic dance.

The risk of accidental injury while walking usually depends on the environment and the setting. Always choose a place to walk that's safe, well-lighted, free of air pollutants, and away from congested traffic (cars, cycles, other pedestrians, and dogs).

A QUICK WAY TO BEAT THE CLOCK

It's a universal truth: Everybody has trouble finding time to exercise. But fitting a walk into a hectic schedule may be easier than you think. If you want to get the most benefit from every minute you exercise, then high-speed walking may be just what you're looking for. If you're ready to pick up the pace, try walking a little faster each day. Instead of walking three miles in 60 minutes, try walking the same distance in 45 minutes. That'll save you some time. For a vigorous exercise program, try race walking, incline walking (on a treadmill), or walking with small hand weights. We'll give you specific ideas and instructions later.

CALORIES *DO* COUNT

If you're not pressed for time, you may be able to burn up more calories by walking. Why? Because walking at a moderate pace increases the possibility of longer, more frequent sessions. Although it can take more time to get the same fitness benefits as jogging or cycling, walking can still result in similar health benefits. These benefits accrue even if you are strolling (20 minutes per mile). Walking burns calories, helps increase HDL levels, and provides some cardiovascular fitness. Look at the chart below to see how many calories you'll burn doing 30 minutes of various activities.

Calories Burned in a 30-Minute Workout

Activity	Body Weight (in lbs.)		
	100	150	200
Walking (2.0 mph or 30 min./mile)	84	120	156
Walking (3.0 mph or 20 min./mile)	112	160	208
Walking (4.5 mph)	154	220	286
Jogging (5.5 mph)	259	370	481
Running (6.0 mph or 10 min./mile)	448	640	832
Swimming (25 yds./min.)	97	138	179
Swimming (50 yds./min.)	175	250	325
Bicycling (6.0 mph or 10 min./mile)	84	120	156
Bicycling (12.0 mph or 5 min./mile)	144	205	267

Note: The more you weigh, the more calories you burn during physical activity, since a heavier body expends more energy.

NO LEARNING CURVE

You already know how to walk. You don't have to learn new skills or take lessons to get started with walking exercise. Aerobic dance, swimming, and racquet sports require a minimum level of skill to participate and to get some benefit. Taking lessons can cost money. And it takes time to become proficient enough to enjoy these activities. Walking is the simplest of all exercises. You can get started and benefit right away.

OTHER REASONS TO WALK: REAL LIFE STORIES

Even if you choose a vigorous exercise like running, you'll probably start out by walking. Many people find it a good idea to make the transition from walking to jogging, and then to running.

 Kathy had been relatively sedentary most of her life. At age 32, she started a physical activity program, walking two miles each morning before work. After about two months, she was able to walk a 15-minute-mile pace comfortably. The results were fantastic. She lost a few pounds and was feeling more energetic than she had in years. It was the first time in her life that Kathy thought of herself as a physically active person.

She enjoyed the activity so much that she decided to pick up the pace a bit and try jogging. She varied the time, walking for 10 minutes, then jogging for 5 minutes, alternating back and forth between walking and jogging for the full 30 minutes. Gradually, she increased the jogging time and decreased the walking. Within a few months she was jogging three miles in 30 minutes. Kathy had made an easy and injury-free transition from being a couch potato to being a jogger.

Walking as a transitional activity can go both ways. People who have been in vigorous, high-impact exercise programs sometimes have had to give up their sport for some reason (such as injury, arthritis, or surgery). Many of these people find that they can get a great workout from walking.

Andy was nearly 60 years old. He had been an avid runner and tennis player most of his adult life. Typically, he jogged twenty miles a week and played three sets of singles tennis two days a week. He was extremely active until he suffered a serious injury in an automobile accident. His doctor said that he'd have to give up jogging and tennis because his lower back couldn't stand the impact.

Andy missed his physical activity and became depressed. He wondered what he could do to keep fit. His physical therapist suggested walking on a treadmill as part of his rehabilitation program. Walking soon became the part of his rehab program that Andy liked the best. When he recovered from his acute injuries, he stayed with the treadmill walking program. Soon he was increasing the incline and walking at a faster pace. This way he achieved the same aerobic intensity as running, but without the impact on his back and joints.

Andy was getting better physically, and he began to feel less depressed. Near the end of the rehab program, Andy began to look for something he could do outdoors. Spring had arrived and he wanted to be outside enjoying it. With his doctor's okay, Andy took up cycling. Andy's transition was easy, because walking uphill worked many of the same leg muscles as cycling did. Andy's recovery was complete.

Walking is also a viable option for people who excel in other physical activities, including elite runners. Runners can walk on "rest" days, walk before or after a race, or even try an occasional hard walk instead of a run.

Craig took his marathon training program seriously. In his program, he varied longer distances (called "hard" days) with shorter distances ("easy" days) as he approached the big event. Walking for some of his training time on the easy days helped his muscles recover from the overload of the hard days. As Craig's hard days got longer, he decided to break up the long distances of running with 5-minute walks. This routine gave him confidence that he could finish the marathon. As he approached the day of the race, he cut back on the intensity of his training. He chose walking instead of running for the last few days before the big race. After the marathon, he decided to lower the intensity of his exercise program by walking instead of running for several days. Walking was a great way for Craig to stay active before he resumed a moderate running program.

Walking is the one physical activity you can adopt as your lifetime exercise program. Or, you can use it as a step to—or from—other fitness activities.

WALKING FOR FUN

Too many people approach exercise with a deadly seriousness. Please, lighten up! Walking is not only good for you, it's fun! Take a look at the list below. It offers a variety of ways to make regular walking a lot less serious. You can try these methods or get creative and come up with your own ideas.

HOW TO PUT MORE FUN INTO WALKING

☐ Walk to different kinds of music. Try marches, classics, even country and western.
☐ Vary your walking route. If you turned right at a corner yesterday, turn left today.
☐ Choose a destination—the store, the library, a friend's house.
☐ Walking gives you time to organize your thoughts. Plan a meal, a party, or your week.
☐ Power walk with weights.
☐ Do interval walking during circuit training.
☐ Wear fun clothes when you walk. Find a wild print shirt, or brightly colored socks. Anything that is cheerful helps make the statement that you're enjoying yourself.
☐ Take a walk in the woods.
☐ Walk backwards sometimes. A word of caution: Try this only on an uncrowded track or other area where the surface is even. Avoid inclines and curbs.
☐ Wave or speak to people you see along the way.
☐ Walk and talk with a child. Try to see the world through young eyes.
☐ _____
☐ _____
☐ _____

If you walk around a track, here's a little trick to help you keep track of the number of laps you have walked. Take along a big handkerchief or a rope or piece of string. Tie a knot in it each time you complete a lap. Count the knots to see how many laps you have walked.

The Classic Rewards of Walking

Walking carries a variety of perks. Some happen almost immediately. Others take a while longer to accrue.

SHORT-TERM BENEFITS

Here are some rewards you can get as soon as you lace up your shoes and start out the door.

- *Walking modifies heart disease risk factors.*

In one study, a group of women walked the same distance every day for twenty-four weeks, but they walked at different speeds ranging from a stroll to a very brisk walk. All groups showed improvements in HDL-cholesterol, the type of blood cholesterol that reduces heart disease risk. So no matter how fast you go, you'll still reap great rewards.

- *Walking helps you make the transition to more vigorous activity.*

If you're out of shape, walking is one exercise you can do at a low intensity. As you become more physically fit, you can gradually increase the frequency, duration, and intensity. You can then "graduate" to more vigorous activities such as brisk walking, jogging, or running, if you want to. Remember, moderate activities also provide health benefits.

- *Walking helps you relax.*

Many people today feel stressed out all the time. Walking is a great way to counteract this stress. When you work your heart and muscles, they relax. And when you're out walking, you can escape from phones, faxes, and beepers for a while. Since walking doesn't require any special skill, you can focus your attention on thinking creatively or problem-solving. Or you can let your mind wander and simply watch the squirrels scamper through crisp leaves, hear the sound of wind in the trees, and smell the roses.

LONG-TERM BENEFITS

As walking becomes a regular habit, over time you can expect to benefit in one or more of the following ways.

- ***Walking reduces your risk of heart disease.***
Walking will reduce your heart disease risk factors, such as high blood cholesterol and high blood pressure.

- ***Walking helps you control your weight.***
If you're overweight, your risk of high blood pressure, high choles- terol, and diabetes increase. And these factors increase the risk of heart disease. Walking burns calories and can help you keep your weight in the normal range. Vacations that include walking or hiking will help counteract the extra meals that are often part of hotel and restaurant dining.

- ***Walking improves the efficiency of your heart and lungs.***
When your heart gets stronger, it doesn't have to work as hard to circulate blood through your body. This puts less strain on your cardiovascular system.

- ***Walking helps keep you physically fit.***
Walking, especially when coupled with strength-building and flexibility activities, can help you stay fit and strong. It helps protect against the natural loss of muscle tone as we age. Instead, you stay stronger longer and can enjoy your "golden years" to the fullest. Many seniors report that their walking program is an important part of their lives. They say it is the key to their enjoyment of travel, vacations, social activities, and family gatherings.

- ***Walking adds to your social life.***
Whether you want to meet other people or just want to spend more time with friends and family, walking can be a time for socializing.

Many worksites and communities have walking groups that are open to all levels, from beginner to race walker. And a walk after dinner is a great way to keep in touch with your spouse or kids.

- *Walking helps you stay active for a lifetime.*
When you were in school, you may have played football, basketball, soccer, or tennis. You may have been a cheerleader or a gymnast. But it's hard to maintain those activities past your twenties and thirties. On the other hand, walking for exercise is easy. It's something you can do well into your sixties, seventies, eighties. . . .

Walking Perks

Put a check beside the benefits of walking that are important to you. Add others that are not listed here.

_____ I already know how to walk. I don't need to learn a new skill.

_____ I don't need to buy any equipment (except walking shoes) or pay any fees.

_____ I can walk with a partner or group.

_____ I can walk alone.

_____ I can walk year-round and in most weather.

_____ I can walk indoors or outdoors.

_____ I can walk for the rest of my life.

_____ I don't need special clothing for walking.

_____ Walking can be a lot of fun.

_____ I can get a good workout through walking.

_____ I can walk for several short bouts or a longer session.

_____ I am more likely to stay with walking than some other forms of exercise.

_____ I don't have to change clothes to walk.

_____ My risk of getting an exercise-related injury while walking is very low.

_____ I can use walking as a transition to or from other more vigorous types of exercise.

_____ Walking will help me achieve significant health benefits.

_____ Walking is a low-impact exercise and is thereby less likely to cause injuries to bones and joints.

_____ There are a lot of places where I can walk.

_____ My walk gives me time to think and solve problems.

_____

_____

_____

_____

Stop Hesitating—Start Motivating

"I just can't seem to make myself exercise."

"I've tried to be active, but I never could keep it up for more than three weeks. I guess I'm just an exercise failure."

These are common statements. People make them every day. But at the American Heart Association, we believe that there's no such thing as an exercise failure. Instead, there are people who simply don't know how to change their sedentary habits into a healthy, active lifestyle.

We've found that these people just need the right techniques and tools to help them embrace physical activity and make it a part of their daily lives. So we've included some useful techniques and tools in this book.

ARE YOU READY OR NOT?

If you're not truly ready to make changes, none of the strategies we talk about here will do you any good. Becoming more active means finding the time, adjusting your lifestyle, and reordering your priorities to make physical activity a regular part of your life, not just another hassle. The quiz on page 26 will help you determine just how ready you are to stop wishing and start walking.

RECORDING YOUR PROGRESS

To change your life, it's important to track your activities, thoughts, and progress. When you put it on paper, you'll learn what situations, people, or places encourage you and which discourage you from being active. Self-monitoring helps you stay on track. And keeping a record of your progress is motivating! On your first day, start using the Walking Diary in Appendix I. Then use it every time you walk. A filled-in sample of the Walking Diary is included and will give you some ideas as to how to keep your own log.

SETTING REASONABLE GOALS

Crusty baseball great Yogi Berra once said, "You've got to be very careful if you don't know where you're going, because you might not get there." He was right! Without goals, it's easy to wander off course. So, set short-term and long-term walking goals that are specific, realistic, and personal. Then follow through. That's the secret to success at anything, including making exercise a part of your life. We'll be helping you develop goals and an action plan for a regular walking program in Chapter 4.

CONTROLLING YOUR "TRIGGERS"

Incidents happen all day long that influence your behavior. They "trigger" a reaction in you. You may be conscious of these triggers, or they can occur subconsciously. When it comes to being physically active, some triggers will encourage you to be active while others may keep you from it.

 Carla planned to walk after work. But when she got home she realized she was feeling worn out after a long, hard day. Besides, she couldn't find her walking shoes right away. To top it off, it started to rain. So she decided not to walk. Instead, she sat in front of the television until it was time to go to bed.

Carla's co-worker, Juan, also planned to walk after work. But just as he was leaving the office, the sky opened up. Juan knew that he couldn't walk in the pouring rain, but he didn't want to miss his walk. Since he kept a pair of walking shoes in the trunk of his car, Juan decided to stop at the shopping mall on his way home. There he finished his 30-minute walk and then took a minute to pick out a small gift for his wife. When he got home, both he and his wife were delighted that Juan had found a way to be active in spite of the rain!

Fatigue and weather conditions are among the most common triggers for inactivity. Triggers are different for each person—they can range from a very long day at work to a disagreement with a family member. Any one of these can potentially throw you off your exercise routine. You need to find out what your triggers are. Then you can plan strategies to eliminate or deal with them when they occur.

WITH A LITTLE HELP FROM YOUR FRIENDS

It's really hard to change your life by yourself. One reason is that the changes you make affect others. For example, if you want to walk right after work, you may need to recruit your spouse to help get dinner on the table. Or you may need company on your walk. Having someone to walk with sometimes makes it more fun and makes the time pass faster.

But if you do decide to change your life, people can support you in many ways. They can participate, provide information, listen while you voice your frustrations, or help you solve problems. You may not need all of these types of support. Nor does one person have to fill all your support needs. First, decide what help you need and who can help you. Then *ask* them for help. Be specific. And don't forget to reward them for their support.

REWARD YOURSELF!

Perhaps you believe that you don't need to reward yourself for being active because it's something you *should* do anyway. When physical activity truly becomes a habit for you, your motivation comes from knowing you are doing something good for yourself. But while you are learning how to make exercise a habit, you may need to find ways that you can reward yourself.

These rewards can be simple—a hot bubble bath, time to read, a night to yourself, a long-distance call to a friend. Or they can be more elaborate—a new suit, a weekend gataway, a vacation, or a new appliance. Tie your rewards to your goals. When you attain a new goal, treat yourself. This will make the process more fun and it will inspire you to continue.

DON'T RUN OUT OF STEAM—WALKING IS A TRIAL RUN

Changing behavior is a process. You will go two steps forward, and one step backward. You will also, on occasion, fall off the exercise wagon.

Michael had been walking 30 minutes, six days a week, for two months. He had lost some weight and was feeling great. A recent checkup showed that his blood pressure level, which had been a little high, was now down in the normal range. He was delighted because it meant he would not have to go on medication.

But then Michael was hit hard with the flu. He was in bed for almost a week. He went back to work the next week but still felt lousy. After two weeks he started walking again, but he was disappointed that he couldn't do the distance or the time he'd been doing. Although he was tempted to throw in the towel, Michael knew that was not the answer. He knew that if he started slow and easy and kept at it, he could get back to his previous level. And keep at it he did. In a month, he was back to his old routine and feeling great.

Michael experienced an unplanned lapse in his walking program. A lapse is a temporary interruption in your program. Lapses happen. In fact, you should count on them happening. The important thing is not to let a lapse lead to a *relapse*. This is when a temporary lapse is dragged out into a longer period of inactivity. A relapse is dangerous because it is one step closer to *collapse*, or totally abandoning your program.

You can prevent lapses and relapses by knowing your triggers. You can also plan ahead for situations that put you at risk of lapsing. For example, staying active during the winter holidays can be difficult. But you can plan to walk in the mall before you begin your holiday shopping. Or you can take a walk (instead of driving) through your neighborhood to see all the lights.

THE POWER OF THINKING POSITIVELY

Keep your attitude upbeat. Your thoughts and internal dialogue greatly influence your actions. Too many people are guilty of "all or nothing" thinking: "If I can't walk every day for the next week, I give up." People also put themselves down when something goes wrong. "I skipped my walk today. I'll never lose the weight. I have no willpower. I'm a failure."

Be aware of how you talk to yourself. Instead of tearing yourself down, try to boost your self-esteem and self-confidence. You'll be more likely to reach your physical activity goals if you do.

These techniques will help you be successful at making walking a habit. All are important. Some will be more helpful than others. And some will be more important at the beginning of your program than later. You'll have a chance to try them out in the next section of this book.

CHAPTER

3

Before You Start

You just bought this book about walking. Congratulations! You're on the right track. Now it's time to put your good intentions to work. You need to be truly psyched up to make walking a part of your lifestyle. It's easy to say, "I've got to get more exercise," but it takes time and energy to put it into action. Making the commitment to make walking a lifetime habit is a big step. That's where this book will help you. You may know someone who just started a walking program and can't stop talking about how great they feel about their new adventure. That's the kind of success you want to have with your walking program. And it may be easier than you think. You've taken the first step by opening this book; now we'll give you ideas to help you make the commitment and stick to it.

Making Your Lifestyle Changes Stick

More and more people are making walking a permanent part of their lifestyle. You may have started a walking program in the past but did not continue. Scientists have found that people who succeed in making permanent lifestyle changes, such as quitting smoking, exercising, or eating less fat, tend to move gradually through a *series* of steps or stages in the process of changing. It seems that progressing slowly through these steps is important to success, because you can't move on to the next step until you've completed the one before.

There are several specific stages you must pass through when you try to make walking (or any other change) a habit. The first thing you need to know is which stage you're in now. Find out by taking this quiz.

The "Are You Ready to Walk?" Quiz

Circle the number that best describes your current situation.

1. I don't presently walk for health or fitness reasons, and have no plans to do so in the next six months.

2. I don't presently walk for health or fitness reasons, but I intend to start soon.

3. I have started walking for health or fitness reasons, but I haven't been able to do it regularly (three or more days per week).

4. I have been walking regularly for health or fitness reasons for less than six months.

5. I have been walking regularly for health or fitness reasons for more than six months *and* I am confident that I can continue my walking program no matter what problems arise.

If you selected #1: At this very early stage, you may not be interested in regular walking for exercise. You may not even know why regular walking would benefit you. Maybe you are concerned about other things going on in your life. Maybe you have a lot of pressure at work or school, or maybe you need to spend more time with the kids. Or maybe you worry about how you'll look in a pair of shorts. If so, you're not alone. But remember, you've got to start somewhere; you've got to crawl before you walk. If you're in this stage, you need to prepare yourself to start thinking about the benefits of a lifetime walking program. Chapter 1 of this book is intended to alert you to the many benefits of being physically active, and it will show you how easy it is to walk for exercise. Take a few minutes to identify *your* reasons for not being active. See the list on pages 2–4.

After you read this chapter, decide if starting a walking program is what you want *right now*. If not, don't beat yourself up! It's better to be honest with yourself than to begin a walking program for the wrong reasons. Start a walking program because it's right for you.

Keep this book handy, then retake "The 'Are You Ready to Walk?'

Quiz" in the next month or two. At some point in the future, you may be truly ready to start a walking program, and this book can help you step off on the right foot.

On the other hand, if you're reading this book, you're probably *not* in the precontemplation stage. The mere fact that you're referring to a book for information on walking shows at least some level of interest.

If you selected #2: You've probably been thinking about walking for exercise for a while. You already know about all the benefits of walking. And you want them for yourself. But for one reason or another, you just haven't been able to do it. Perhaps you don't know whether it's safe for you to start walking. Maybe you don't know how to pick a good pair of walking shoes. Or you just don't think you have the time. Some people get stuck in this stage for a while before moving on.

But this book can help you. It will help you set goals, choose the right equipment, start at the right level, and stay motivated. The main thing you need to remember is to start off gradually and allow yourself the time to adjust so that walking becomes a regular part of your lifestyle.

If you selected #3: You've walked a bit to stay fit and healthy, but you can't seem to keep it up for more than a couple of days or weeks. You know the benefits, you have the desire, and you know how to do it. You just need help to make walking a *regular* part of your life.

If you're in this stage, you need to identify any barriers that keep you from walking regularly. Weather, boredom, illness, injury, and vacations are some of the more common excuses that people have for relapsing into their sedentary ways. It's important to find out what your barriers are and then plan ways around them. Be sure to read the sections on goal-setting (Chapter 5), monitoring your success (Chapter 8), balancing your fitness program (Chapter 10), and special opportunities to walk (Chapter 14). These should help you become a more consistent walker.

If you selected #4: Congratulations! You've been able to maintain a regular walking program. Feels pretty good, doesn't it? You're in what scientists call the "action stage." That's because you're *taking action* to incorporate walking into your life. Even so, you may have some nagging concerns about being able to sustain it for the rest of your life.

The action stage is dynamic. Chances are you've experienced one or more setbacks or lapses. Perhaps you even stopped walking for a couple of days or even a week. Lapses are a natural part of learning how to maintain a habit. Think of toddlers who fall half a dozen times in an afternoon. They'll sit there for a moment, but then they pick themselves up and keep going. Likewise, you need to know how to keep a simple lapse from becoming a more dangerous relapse. A severe relapse might set you back into the preparation or contemplation stages.

This book has several features to help keep you on track. For example, you may want to vary your walking by adding some advanced walking techniques (Chapter 9). The diary at the back of the book will help you keep track of your goals and progress. There are tips for preventing relapse on pages 93–95. And don't forget to reward yourself (pages 91–92). Also, we'll show you how to look for opportunities to be active on vacations, in your community, or in another city.

If you selected #5: Everyone who ever laced up a walking shoe wants to be able to stick with it for life. You found a way to do it. Most importantly, you know how to stay active despite the inevitable bad weather, illness, family emergencies, work commitments, and vacations. Chances are you are reaping many of the benefits listed on pages 1–2.

But don't throw away this book! It can still help you sharpen some of your walking and physical activity skills and will give you opportunities to set new goals and challenges and learn new techniques. Share your ideas and experiences with friends or family members who can use them in their efforts to become physically active. Keep up the good work!

Are You Ready?

For most people, starting a walking program is completely safe. If you start gradually, there should be little if any muscle soreness; you probably won't experience any physical symptoms at all. Starting slowly can also help you reduce the risk of injury.

However, if it has been a while since you were active on a regular basis, or if you're a man over 40 or a woman over 50, you might want to see your doctor before you start a serious walking program. The following checklist can help you decide.

Do I Need a Medical Okay?

Mark the items that apply to you:

___ You have a heart condition and your doctor recommends only medically supervised physical activity.

___ During or right after you exercise, you frequently have pains or pressure in the left or mid-chest area, left neck, shoulder, or arm.

___ You have developed chest pain within the last month.

___ You tend to lose consciousness or fall over due to dizziness.

___ You feel extremely breathless after mild exertion.

___ Your doctor recommended that you take medicine for high blood pressure or a heart condition.

___ You have bone or joint problems.

___ You have a medical condition or other physical reason not mentioned here that might need special attention in an exercise program (such as insulin-dependent diabetes).

___ You are a male over age 40 or a female over age 50, have not been physically active, and are planning a relatively *vigorous* walking program.

Note: This checklist was developed from several sources, particularly the Physical Activity Readiness Questionnaire, British Columbia Ministry of Health, Department of National Health and Welfare, Canada (revised 1992).

If you checked one or more items, see your doctor before you start walking. Chances are, he or she can help you create a walking plan that meets your special needs.

If you didn't check any items, feel free to start a gradual, sensible walking program anytime.

If you feel any of the physical symptoms listed above when you start your walking program, contact your doctor right away.

How Fit Are You Now?

Before you can determine what walking program is best for you, it's important to know your current fitness level. Are you a complete couch potato? Are you active on the job? (That can give you a head start.) Are you already physically active?

The following easy, one-mile walking test will give you a general idea of your current fitness level. Take this test only if you're not taking blood pressure medicine, heart or lung medicine, antidepressants, drugs to help you lose weight, or any other drug that lowers or raises your heart rate. This test will not be valid if you're using these medicines.

Before you take this fitness test, make sure you've completed the "Do I Need A Medical Okay?" questionnaire on page 29. If you experience any unusual pain or discomfort during any part of the test, STOP IMMEDIATELY and consult your doctor.

Preparing for the Test

- Don't drink caffeinated beverages (coffee, tea, colas) or eat a heavy meal for at least three hours before the test.
- Find a measured, one-mile track at a school, park, or recreation center. If you want to measure your own course, make sure it has a good surface and no hills.
- Take a stopwatch or a watch with a second hand, a pencil or pen, and this book with you to the track. Wear comfortable walking shoes.
- Don't do the test outdoors when it is extremely hot, cold, or windy. Your time and exercising heart rate may not be valid under these conditions.
- Practice taking your pulse before doing this test. (See page 43 for more information and illustrations.)
- Walk a few minutes to warm up before starting the test.

TAKING THE TEST

Start walking as quickly as you can to get your heart rate up to at least 110 beats per minute without straining. You should be able to talk while walking. To check your heart rate at your neck or wrist, count the number of pulse beats in 10 seconds and multiply by 6. This will give you the beats per minute. For example, if you count 20 beats in 10 seconds, your heart rate is 120 beats per minute. (For information on how to properly calculate your heart rate, see pages 42-45.)

Measure your pulse 5 minutes into your walk. Make sure your pulse is up to at least 110 beats per minute. Keep a constant pace, and keep your breathing smooth and regular. If you are too winded to talk, slow down.

As soon as you cross the one-mile mark, check the time in minutes and seconds that it took you to walk the mile. (Most people take between 10 and 20 minutes to walk this distance.) Slow your pace, but keep moving. Immediately take your pulse. On the Personal Data Record sheet in Appendix III, write down your total time and your finishing heart rate in the section marked "Baseline." There is room for you to put other health information in this chart as well. Continue to walk slowly for 3 to 5 minutes to allow your heart rate and blood pressure to return to normal levels.

SCORING YOUR TEST

Locate the chart for Scoring the One-Mile Fitness Test in Appendix II. Find your age group and your heart rate. If your exact pulse isn't shown, round it off to the nearest 10 beats.

Now read across the times listed for men and women in columns A and B.

- ☐ If the time it took you to walk the mile *was between the times listed in columns A and B,* you're in the *moderate fitness* category.
- ☐ If your time for the walking test was *the same as for column A or it took you longer* to walk the mile, you are in the *low fitness* category.
- ☐ If your time for the walking test was *the same as in column B or it took you less time,* you're in the *high fitness* category.

 Stephen is a 52-year-old man. He walked the one-mile course in 15 minutes. His finishing heart rate was 130 beats per minute. Stephen is in the moderate fitness level. This is what his baseline record looks like.

| | One-Mile Fitness Test | | | | | | | |
Interval	Date	Time	Heart Rate	Fitness Category	Body Weight	Blood Pressure	Blood Cholesterol	Other
Baseline	10/23	15:00	130	Moderate				
One Month								
Two Months								
Three Months								

Janet is a 43-year-old woman. She walked the mile in 17 minutes and 50 seconds with a finishing heart rate of 140 beats per minute. Janet is in the low fitness level category.

| | One-Mile Fitness Test | | | | | | | |
Interval	Date	Time	Heart Rate	Fitness Category	Body Weight	Blood Pressure	Blood Cholesterol	Other
Baseline	3/16	17:50	140	Low				
One Month								
Two Months								
Three Months								

Of course, this test is just a rough estimate of your actual fitness. But it *is* a place to start. After about four weeks of regular walking, test yourself again to check your progress. Record your results in the Personal Data Record in Appendix III. Over time, you'll see a change: You will cover the mile faster or your heart rate will be lower when you finish. These are both sure signs that your fitness level is improving.

You might want to take the one-mile test a couple of times a year to make sure that you're still improving. Continue to record your results in the space provided in Appendix III.

An alternative to taking the one-mile fitness test is to simply time how long it takes you to walk one mile. Repeat the timed walk once a month for three to six months to monitor your progress. Walking the same distance in a faster time means you are becoming more physically fit.

Another easy way to measure fitness is to see how far you can walk in 20 minutes. After a month or two of regular walking, go for another 20-minute test walk and see how far you go. If you are able to walk farther than the first time, your fitness level has improved. This test is especially useful for people who do not have a measured one-mile track or route.

The Many Faces of Walking

Walking may seem like a pretty simple thing. And at face value, it really is. But actually, there are several types of walking. As you begin to plan your walking program, you may find that you need to start with one type of walking, then gradually build to another.

STROLLING

Strolling is the type of walking that people do most of the time. Typically, when you're strolling, you don't increase your heart or breathing rates very much. It's a comfortable pace that's typically interrupted by frequent stops. Shopping and vacation sightseeing are examples of strolling.

Strolling is easy to do. You don't have to change clothes, you don't sweat, and you can often fit it in while you're doing other things. Strolling may give you some health and feel-good benefits, but it won't boost your cardiovascular fitness. However, it's a good way to start on an exercise program.

If your score on the one-mile fitness test put you in the low fitness category, you may want to begin your exercise program by spending more time strolling. Even short bouts of strolling are better than being sedentary. Your goal is to increase your walking time. For example:

Instead of . . .	
Watching TV	Take a walk at a nearby nature center, park, or arboretum.
Sitting through TV commercials	Get up and walk around the house.
Taking a bus tour	Find a walking tour of the same sights.
Walking the dog for only a few minutes	Extend the walk for 10 or 15 minutes (your dog probably needs the exercise, too!).

Make it your goal to walk more often. As your fitness level improves, you can begin a more vigorous fitness walking program.

PURPOSEFUL WALKING

You're late for the bus so you pick up your pace. Or you're trying to keep up with your three-year-old on her new tricycle. These are examples of purposeful walking. In these instances, you probably find that you breathe heavier and your heart rate picks up a little. That's a sign that your heart and lungs are having to work harder. As a result, you are more likely to get health and fitness benefits from purposeful walking than from strolling.

Like strolling, an advantage of purposeful walking is that it's usually tied to another activity. That way you don't feel as if you're working out. This is especially important if you don't see yourself as a jock or can't seem to find a block of time during the day to change clothes and work out. But as with strolling, the best way to get benefits from purposeful walking is by finding ways to fit it into your normal day, every day. For example:

Instead of . . .	
Parking right at the door	Park further from your office or shopping mall.
Letting your dog stay in the back yard	Walk your dog every day.
Sitting in the bleachers	Walk around the playing field at your kids' sports games.
Riding the bus right to your front door	Get off the bus sooner and walk the rest of the way.
Ordering lunch in or getting in your car to go out to eat	Walk to a nearby restaurant for lunch.

If you're in the low or moderate fitness category and want to begin a more structured walking program, purposeful walking is a good place to start. As you begin to build more walking into your day, you'll want to find other ways to improve your walking and your fitness level.

FITNESS WALKING

If you're at the moderate or high fitness level, you may want to start with fitness walking. This means walking at a pace that really challenges your heart and lungs. To improve your fitness level, you'll need to walk at a brisk pace for at least 30 minutes, three to five days a week.

Because of this faster pace, there will be more impact on your joints than with less strenuous types of walking. For that reason, you'll need proper walking shoes (see pages 57–62).

The benefits of fitness walking are numerous. Your heart and lungs work more efficiently, you burn more calories at a faster rate, and you'll likely see results sooner than with less rigorous walking.

Still, if you're not able to start out at this level, that's okay. It is better to start with purposeful walking, and then build your fitness level gradually.

ADVANCED WALKING

Believe it or not, there is an *advanced* level of walking.

Have you ever watched the race walkers compete during the Olympics? They're the ones who look so funny, with their arms and hips going in all sorts of directions as they race around the track. Advanced walking requires a high level of fitness. It also requires special techniques and equipment. Advanced walkers may use hand weights. They may also walk on a treadmill positioned at a steep incline or use hills, bridges, or stairs for a more grueling workout.

This type of walking is not for everyone. It's especially not for people who are just starting a walking program. But if you're already physically fit and want to maintain or even boost your fitness level, advanced walking is a great way to do it. It can also help you by adding variety to your walking, which can keep you interested and challenged. If you like to compete, walking at this level allows you to participate in walking races. Check to see if there is a walking club in your community. For more information on advanced walking, see Chapter 9.

CHAPTER

4

F.I.T.T. for Life

Choosing the Right Walking Plan

You're fully committed to the active way of life. You also know your current fitness level and you've read about the different types of walking. Now, let's build a customized walking plan just for you.

To design a walking plan, you can choose from a couple of different approaches. One of them may work better for you than the other, so you decide. But, most importantly, remember that you can always change your plan as your fitness level or walking interests change.

STRICTLY TRADITIONAL—THE EXERCISE APPROACH

Okay. You want to improve the strength and efficiency of your heart and lungs. You do that by training them to do more than they're used to. To get this conditioning effect, exercise scientists have traditionally recommended a program that includes the following elements. They're easy to remember because they spell "F.I.T.T."—which is what you want to be.

THE TRADITIONAL F.I.T.T. FORMULA
☐ Frequency—three to five times per week
☐ Intensity—50 percent to 85 percent of maximal heart rate (i.e., moderate to vigorous intensity)

☐ Time—at least 20 to 30 continuous minutes per exercise session

☐ Type—aerobic activities (jogging, bicycling, swimming, walking)

You can personalize this F.I.T.T. formula based on your physical activity interests and fitness level. For example, if you haven't exercised in a long time or your fitness level is low, you'll want to start out at the lower levels of each F.I.T.T. element. As your fitness level improves, you can gradually increase the frequency, intensity, and time. An example of a beginning walking program using the traditional approach would be:

Monday	Walk 20 minutes at 55 percent target heart rate
Tuesday	Rest
Wednesday	Walk 20 minutes at 55 percent target heart rate
Thursday	Rest
Friday	Rest
Saturday	Walk 20 minutes at 55 percent target heart rate
Sunday	Rest

This traditional F.I.T.T. formula has been used for decades to help people boost fitness and cut their risk of heart disease, high blood pressure, and diabetes. In recent years, scientists have developed another approach to help Americans get off that couch. Consider both approaches and choose the one that seems right for you.

THE "WORKED IN" WORKOUT—
A LIFESTYLE APPROACH

The number one reason most people give for not getting enough exercise is lack of time. Even 20 to 30 minutes three times a week may be too difficult for some people. Other people aren't ready for a vigorous exercise program such as running. "Easy does it" is their motto.

The good news: Recent research has found that people who are moderately active on a regular basis get many of the same health benefits as those who work out more vigorously. These benefits include improved blood cholesterol levels, weight loss, and a reduced risk of heart disease. In other words, just do *something*. Health experts are recommending a lifestyle-oriented approach that includes the following features:

LIFESTYLE F.I.T.T. FORMULA

□ Frequency—most days, preferably every day

□ Intensity—moderate (equivalent to 15- to 20-minute-per-mile pace)

□ Time—accumulate at least 30 minutes per day; does not have to be continuous

□ Type—any aerobic activity including lifestyle activities like vacuuming, gardening, walking, etc.

We call this the "Lifestyle" approach because it allows you to count many of your day-to-day activities as exercise. These activities include housework, yard work, or purposeful walking. To count as exercise, these activities must be done regularly and at a moderate level of intensity. The lifestyle approach also permits greater flexibility, allowing you to fit physical activity into your daily routine. And if you're out of shape or dislike sports, the lifestyle approach gives you an exercise alternative.

A one-week example of a lifestyle walking program is:

Monday	Walk the dog for 10 minutes; two 5-minute walks at the office; 15-minute walk at lunch
Tuesday	Walk the dog for 10 minutes; a 10-minute walk at the office vacuum carpets for 15 minutes
Wednesday	Walk the dog for 10 minutes; two 5-minute walks at office; 15-minute walk at lunch
Thursday	Walk at mall for 15 minutes at lunch; walk to client's office and back for 20 minutes
Friday	Rest
Saturday	Walk the dog for 15 minutes; rake leaves for 25 minutes
Sunday	Walk at park with family for 30 minutes; dig in flower beds for 90 minutes

TRADITIONAL OR LIFESTYLE: WHICH IS RIGHT FOR YOU?

We found out long ago that a single approach to exercise doesn't work for everyone. Some people prefer a traditional exercise program.

They want to get fit, and they want it now. Others like the lifestyle approach. This way, they can work physical activity into their day naturally, without disturbing their daily routine. The lifestyle approach may also work for people who travel. They can fit in a walk between flights while waiting in the terminal. Some people like to combine the two approaches. For example, they may be able to do a couple of days of traditional walking on the weekends and work in three to five days of lifestyle walking during the week.

Remember, regardless of the walking approach you choose, both can:

☐ reduce blood pressure levels
☐ contribute to weight loss
☐ reduce blood cholesterol levels
☐ make you feel good

Each approach has its own advantages and disadvantages, too. Let's first take a look at a few of the advantages that are unique to either the traditional or lifestyle approach.

ADVANTAGES

Traditional	*Lifestyle*
■ Strengthens heart and lungs	■ Doesn't usually require changing clothes
■ Can be done all at once	
■ May result in improved fitness more quickly	■ Can be done in many short bouts throughout the day
	■ Can be a good starting point for people who have not exercised in a long time

Here are a few of the disadvantages that are unique to each approach.

DISADVANTAGES

Traditional	*Lifestyle*
■ Requires a 20-plus-minute block of time	■ Only strengthens heart and lungs if done regularly and at a moderate or higher level

- May require special equipment or skills
- May require showering and changing clothes

- Level of intensity may be too hard for people who are out of shape

- Requires creativity to find many ways during the day to be active
- May require a more conscious effort to walk several times during the day
- Level of intensity may not be satisfying for people who are fit

Look carefully at the pros and cons of each approach. Then determine which one will work best for you. If you still aren't sure, consider your current fitness level and your walking readiness.

Remember: You don't have to stay with one approach for the rest of your life. For example, you might want to start out doing lifestyle activities. When you build up enough fitness, you can launch a more traditional program, or vice versa. Consider Paul's story.

 An avid fitness walker, Paul made sure he walked briskly for at least 40 minutes, five days a week. But as a tax accountant, he found it difficult to keep up his walking program in the early spring. To prevent losing most of his fitness during this busy time, he tried to include more walking during his regular day. He parked further from the office and walked in, took the stairs to the printer on the next floor, and walked with his family on the weekends. When tax season was over, Paul switched back to his traditional walking program, gradually increasing it to former levels.

How Often Should You Walk?

First, look at your current fitness level, then at your approach to walking. Those answers may help you determine the number of days per week you want to walk. In general, the more fit you are, the more days you'll want to walk. Of course, if you're using the lifestyle approach, you'll need to walk on most days, regardless of your fitness level. Use the table below to help you decide the right frequency at which to start.

Current Fitness Level	Traditional Approach (days per week)	Lifestyle Approach (days per week)
Low	3–5	4–5
Moderate	4–5	5–7
High	4–6	*

*You may not be able to maintain a high fitness level with a lifestyle walking program.

Remember, it's best to start out walking at the lower end of the range cited for each fitness category. Then you can gradually increase the number of days you walk.

How Should You Pace Your Walks?

You're walking for fitness, right? So you must make sure you're walking fast enough to give you these health benefits. At the same time, you don't want to go so fast that you tire quickly or cause injury. To tell if you are walking at your best pace, use the following methods.

THE TALK TEST

The easiest method for gauging your workout's intensity is the Talk Test. And it's simply this:

- ☐ If you can talk fairly easily while walking, you're doing okay.
- ☐ If you can sing, you need to step up the pace a little.
- ☐ If you can't talk, slow down—you're working too hard!

This super-easy method is ideal for lifestyle-oriented walking where you walk often, but perhaps not at a level that gets your heart rate in the target zone (see below). It also doesn't require any special skills or equipment.

RATING OF PERCEIVED EXERTION

Here's another easy way to help gauge the intensity of your walks. All you do is label how hard the workout feels. Use the Perceived Exertion Scale below to describe your sense of effort. For example, if you are walking at a comfortable pace but you are aware that your heart rate has increased slightly, you might rate the effort as a 1 or a

2. If you're gasping for breath and feel tired all over, you might rate your effort as an 8, 9, or 10.

If your fitness level is low or if you haven't exercised in a while, you'll probably want to keep your Rating of Perceived Exertion (RPE) at 2 or 3. Then gradually work your way up to walking at an RPE between 3 and 6.

The advantage of this method is that you don't have to learn how to take your heart rate or interrupt your walk to measure it.

	Perceived Exertion Scale
0	No perceptible change
1	Very light
2	Light
3	Moderate
4	Somewhat strong
5	Strong
6	↓
7	Very strong
8	
9	↓
10	Very, very strong (almost maximal)
*	Maximal effort

TARGET HEART RATE

When you're walking, there is another way to tell if you are working out at the right level. It's called your target heart rate zone. How does it work? You begin by taking your pulse at different times during your walk. Why? Because as your workout intensity increases, your heart beats faster. How fast should it beat during your walk? That depends, first of all, on your *maximum* heart rate. This rate is the fastest your heart can beat. The rate naturally decreases with age. You can calculate your maximum heart rate by subtracting your current age from 220. For example, if you are 50, your maximum heart rate is about 170 (220–50 = 170). How does that relate to the target heart rate? Your target heart rate is a percentage of your maximum heart rate.

Unless you're in excellent condition, it's too strenuous to exercise above 75 percent of your maximum heart rate. On the other hand, exercising below 50 percent of your maximum heart rate won't adequately condition your heart and lungs. So, you want to aim for between 50 and 75 percent of your maximum heart rate. This 50 to 75 percent range is called target heart rate zone. See the table on page 44 to find your appropriate target zone.

To find out if you are in your target heart rate zone, you'll have to take your pulse several times during your workout, and immediately after you stop exercising. Here's how to do it:

1. Keep moving as you quickly place the tips of the first two fingers of one hand lightly over one of the main blood vessels on your neck (carotid arteries). These arteries are located to the left and right of your Adam's apple. Another convenient place is the inside of your wrist, just below the base of your thumb.

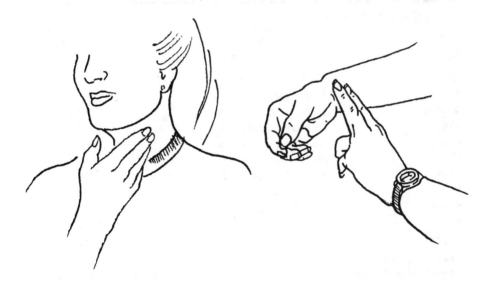

2. Count your pulse for 10 seconds and multiply by 6.
3. If your pulse falls within your target zone, you're doing fine. If it's below your target zone, walk a little faster. If you're above your target zone, slow down. Don't try to exercise at your maximum heart rate—that's working too hard!

The next step is to use the Target Heart Rate Table below to find your target zone. Simply find your age and read the line across. For example, if you're 38, the closest age on the chart is 40; your target zone is 90 to 135 beats per minute.

As you become more fit, you can work up to exercising at higher levels, say 85 percent of your maximum heart rate. To do this with walking, you may have to use advanced walking techniques such as walking uphill, carrying light hand weights, or race walking. (See Chapter 9 for more information.)

HELPFUL TIPS

- Practice taking your pulse until you can do it quickly.
- When you know how it feels to be walking within your target zone, check your pulse to make sure you are exercising at the right level. At least once each week during the first three months and periodically after that, check your pulse as you walk.

Target Heart Rate Table*

Age	Target HR Zone 50–75% of Maximum	Average Maximum Heart Rate
20 years	100–150 beats per minute	200
25 years	98–146 beats per minute	195
30 years	95–142 beats per minute	190
35 years	93–138 beats per minute	185
40 years	90–135 beats per minute	180
45 years	88–131 beats per minute	175
50 years	85–127 beats per minute	170
55 years	83–123 beats per minute	165
60 years	80–120 beats per minute	160
65 years	78–116 beats per minute	155
70 years	75–113 beats per minute	150

*These figures are averages and should be used as general guidelines.
Note: A few high blood pressure medicines lower the maximum heart rate and thus the target zone rate. If you are taking a high blood pressure medication, call your doctor to find out if you should adjust your exercise program.

PUTTING IT ALL TOGETHER

How do you decide which assessment method is best for you? In general, if you're following a traditional approach to walking, use either the target heart rate or RPE method. For the lifestyle approach, use the RPE or the talk test. You may want to use all of these methods. If you start with the Talk Test but find out you're always unable to talk and walk at the same time, the target heart rate is very helpful. With these assessment tools, you can now evaluate the intensity of your walking program. Just use the approach that is right for you and the assessment method you like best. Then use the chart below to help you determine the intensity level.

Workout Intensity Table

Current Fitness Level	Traditional Approach	Lifestyle Approach
Low	50–60% of maximum heart rate or RPE of 3–6	RPE of 3–6 or Talk Test
Moderate	55–75% of maximum heart rate or RPE of 4–9	RPE of 4–9 or Talk Test
High	65–85% of maximum heart rate or RPE of 6–10	*

*You may not be able to maintain a high fitness level using a lifestyle walking program.

How Long Should You Walk?

Are you going to use the traditional or lifestyle approach? The one you choose will determine how long you should walk. With the traditional approach, you do all of your exercising at once. With the lifestyle approach, you'll probably be exercising in many short sessions each day. But in both cases, you need to start at a low level and gradually build up your total time.

Walking Time

Current Fitness Level	Traditional Approach	Lifestyle Approach
Low	5–30 minutes	Accumulate 10–30 minutes (e.g., six 2-minute walks)
Moderate	10–30 minutes	Accumulate at least 30 minutes (e.g., six 5-minute walks)
High	20–45 + minutes	*

*You may not be able to maintain a high fitness level using a lifestyle walking program.

A Customized Walking Plan

Now that you have chosen all of the parts of your walking program, complete the walking plan below. In the next chapter, we'll talk about how to make it happen.

My F.I.T.T. Walking Plan

Frequency _____

Intensity _____

Time _____

Type _____
(Traditional, Lifestyle, or Combination)

SAMPLE TRADITIONAL WALKING PROGRAMS

One the following pages we have given you three different sample walking programs, one for every fitness level. Within each program, you should start at an easy level. Gains in fitness are obtained gradually by slowly increasing the time spent walking and the number of days walked each week. Program A is designed for people in the low fitness category. Program B will help people in the moderate fitness category improve their fitness level. For people already in the high fitness category, Program C is appropriate. Note that each program includes a warm-up and a cool-down period. During these periods you should continue to walk but more slowly.

Program A

	Warm-up	Target Zone Exercising	Cool-down	Frequency Per Week
Week 1	5 min.	5 min.	5 min.	3
Week 2	5 min.	7 min.	5 min.	3
Week 3	5 min.	9 min.	5 min.	3–4
Week 4	5 min.	11 min.	5 min.	3–4
Week 5	5 min.	13 min.	5 min.	3–4
Week 6	5 min.	15 min.	5 min.	3–4
Week 7	5 min.	18 min.	5 min.	3–4
Week 8	5 min.	20 min.	5 min.	3–4

	Warm-up	Target Zone Exercising	Cool-down	Frequency Per Week
Week 9	5 min.	23 min.	5 min.	3–5
Week 10	5 min.	26 min.	5 min.	3–5
Week 11	5 min.	28 min.	5 min.	3–5
Week 12	5 min.	30 min.	5 min.	3–5

Week 13 and on: Check your level of intensity (using the Talk Test, Rating of Perceived Exertion, or exercise pulse rate) periodically to see if you are walking within your target zone. As you become more fit, try exercising within the upper range of your target zone. Gradually increase your brisk walking time to 30 to 60 minutes, at least three times a week. Remember that while your goal is to build your cardiovascular fitness, you also want to have fun!

Program B

	Warm-up	Target Zone Exercising	Cool-down	Frequency Per Week
Week 1	5 min.	10 min.	5 min.	3
Week 2	5 min.	12 min.	5 min.	3–4
Week 3	5 min.	15 min.	5 min.	3–4
Week 4	5 min.	20 min.	5 min.	3–4
Week 5	5 min.	22 min.	5 min.	3–4
Week 6	5 min.	25 min.	5 min.	3–4
Week 7	5 min.	27 min.	5 min.	3–4
Week 8	5 min.	32 min.	5 min.	3–4
Week 9	5 min.	34 min.	5 min.	3–5
Week 10	5 min.	36 min.	5 min.	3–5
Week 11	5 min.	40 min.	5 min.	3–5
Week 12	5 min.	42 min.	5 min.	3–5

Week 13 and on: Check your level of intensity (using the Talk Test, Rating of Perceived Exertion, or exercise pulse rate) periodically to see if you are walking within your target zone. As you become more fit, try exercising within the upper range of your target zone. Gradually increase your brisk walking time to at least 40 minutes, at least three times a week.

Program C

	Warm-up	Target Zone Exercising	Cool-down	Frequency Per Week
Week 1	5 min.	20 min.	5 min.	3–4
Week 2	5 min.	22 min.	5 min.	3–4
Week 3	5 min.	25 min.	5 min.	3–4
Week 4	5 min.	30 min.	5 min.	3–4
Week 5	5 min.	32 min.	5 min.	4–5
Week 6	5 min.	35 min.	5 min.	4–5
Week 7	5 min.	37 min.	5 min.	4–5
Week 8	5 min.	40 min.	5 min.	4–5
Week 9	5 min.	42 min.	5 min.	4–5 +
Week 10	5 min.	45 min.	5 min.	4–5 +
Week 11	5 min.	50 min.	5 min.	4–5 +
Week 12	5 min.	55 min.	5 min.	4–5 +

Week 13 and on: Check your level of intensity (using the Talk Test, Rating of Perceived Exertion, or exercise pulse rate) periodically to see if you are walking within your target zone. As you become more fit, try exercising within the upper range of your target zone. Maintain your brisk walking time at least 55 minutes, at least four times a week.

5

On Your Mark!

Setting Goals

No walking program just happens. You have to work to make it happen. Setting your goals, identifying barriers, planning your approach, acting on your plans, and measuring your progress are all essential to making your regular walking program a reality.

Of course, there are as many ways to set goals as there are people to set them. The key is finding ways that work for you. Chances are, you're not in the habit of setting goals. Most people aren't. But it's a critical element for success in making any change.

Start with what you want to accomplish. Are you walking to boost your energy, lose weight, get in shape for a five-kilometer fun walk, or reduce your risk of heart disease? Maybe you have multiple goals. The first step in setting goals is deciding what you want. If you have more than one goal, first pick the one that is most important to you.

Your success in achieving your goals will reflect how realistic you were in setting them as well as how much you personally want to achieve those goals. Don't try to achieve goals other people set for you unless those goals are really important to you.

LONG- AND SHORT-RANGE GOALS

Nobody runs a marathon the first time they start running. Instead, they first set their long-range goal of running the marathon. Then they set a series of short-range goals: first, to run around the block, then one mile, then five miles, ten miles, and fifteen miles. You get the picture. Walking for fitness is no different. You need a long-range goal and several short-range ones.

SETTING YOUR LONG-RANGE GOAL

Your long-range goals are objectives you want to attain in six months, a year, or even longer. Some people have a specific long-range goal. For example:

"In one year, I want to be able to walk 60 minutes without stopping and without feeling it the next day."

Long-range goals, however, don't have to be specific and detailed. For example:

"In one year, I want to have increased my fitness level with a traditional walking program."

Your long-range goals must be flexible enough to take advantage of unexpected opportunities. You may also have to adjust to unanticipated difficulties. For example:

"Since the baby arrived, I am having difficulty fitting in my 30-minute-a-day walking workouts. Instead, my goal is to walk for 20 to 30 minutes on four or more days."

Your outlook and values may change over time.

"I find a traditional walking program difficult to follow. Instead, my goal is to maintain my fitness level by getting in a total of at least 40 minutes of moderate lifestyle activities on most days."

SETTING YOUR SHORT-RANGE GOALS

Essentially, short-range goals are steps toward accomplishing your long-range goal. In other words, they're sub-goals.

"To improve my fitness level, I want to increase my walking time to at least 30 minutes on at least three days per week for the next two months."

Short-range goals can also be simple goals that don't take a lot of time, energy, or effort to attain.

"To boost the probability of starting my walking program, I will purchase a new pair of comfortable shoes by the end of next week."

It's critical to set both long- and short-range goals. The long-range goals help you focus on what you want. That's especially important if roadblocks tend to sidetrack you. Short-range goals help you experience quick and frequent success. And we all know that there's nothing like success to keep you motivated!

Take some time now to think about your long- and short-range walking goals.

Long-Range Goals

> _____
> _____
> _____

Short-Range Goals

> _____
> _____
> _____
> _____
> _____
> _____

DEFINING A GOAL

Reaching your goal successfully comes from choosing a good goal and stating it correctly. Look at the goals you listed above and check to see if they pass the following tests:

- ### *Is this a goal I want to accomplish?*

Do *I* want it, or am I doing it for someone else? Or because I "should"? Or because someone else told me I must? Truly owning a goal means that *you* are committed to the goal. That kind of commitment and readiness will help keep you motivated during rough times.

- ### *Is my goal specific?*

As we said, long-range goals must be somewhat flexible to accommodate unanticipated events or changes in our values over time, but they must also be specific. This is important to setting achievable long-range goals, and it is *essential* for setting short-range goals. For a goal to be specific, it must include answers to the following questions:

- ☐ What specifically do I want to have happen?
- ☐ When do I want it to happen?
- ☐ How will I know when I have it? (Do I have ways to measure goal attainment, including periodic checkpoints for assessing progress?)

For example, instead of, "I want to improve my fitness level," (non-specific, no "due date," no assessment) a better goal statement would be: "I want to improve from the low to the moderate fitness category on the one-mile walking test in sixteen weeks. To accomplish this I will walk briskly at least five days per week, working up to at least 30 minutes per session."

- ### *Is my goal realistic?*

Your goals should be challenging but attainable. Defeat or failure can take the wind right out of your sails, so it's much better to set a goal that's easier rather than harder. At the same time, you must be somewhat challenged in order to grow. For example, it's more realistic to say, "I will walk for 30 minutes at least three days a week for the next three months" than "I will walk for 30 minutes seven days a week for the next three months."

Review the goals you listed on page 51. Are they clearly defined, specific, and realistic? If you want to, rewrite them.

What! More Barriers?

Unfortunately, yes. Barriers are always in the picture. In fact, you'll face them every step of the way. That's why you have to go at them aggressively. Here's what we mean.

When you're confident that each goal you listed above is truly your own, is specific, and is realistic, you must ask yourself, "What's stopping me from attaining this goal now?" Another way to say that is, "What roadblocks are standing in my way?" Roadblocks usually fall into the following categories discussed below.

LACK OF KNOWLEDGE

Sometimes you simply don't have the information you need to attain your goal. For example, you may not know which shoes are best for walking. This roadblock is easy. You can hurdle it by asking experts, reading, taking a walking class, or attending a seminar. In fact, this book will help you learn about walking shoes, as well as everything else you need to know about starting a walking program.

LACK OF SKILLS

Let's say you know how to start a walking program. The trouble is, you don't know how to apply what you know. With a little effort and attention, you can pass this roadblock by getting some hands-on training, watching other walkers, and practicing to build your skills.

You may know a little about walking. But you need to seek help from other sources in order to learn new skills. Of course, whenever you learn something new, you need to practice it often or you're likely to forget it.

LACK OF SOCIAL SUPPORT

Let's say you know about walking and you have the skills you need. But the people around you don't support your efforts. This lack of support can make attaining your goals difficult.

As we have mentioned, supportive family, friends, neighbors, and social groups can help you reach your walking goals. They can offer words of encouragement, help you gather information, walk with you, or simply listen to your concerns and problems without judging.

But to get this kind of help, you have to ask for it. And, like many people, you may be reluctant to do so. Or it may be that you don't want to impose on others. But you *need* support from the people in your life! To get that help, first find out what kind of support you need. Then determine who can help you. Remember, tell each one what you need. Then, after they help you, be sure to show your appreciation.

UNWILLINGNESS TO TAKE RISKS

"Nothing ventured, nothing gained," the old saying goes. But many people are so afraid of failing that they don't even *try*. The truth is, all of life is a risk. If a given effort works out, great! If not, you've probably learned something from the experience. If you have the feeling that it's safer to stay where you are than to risk making a change, it's time to take a hard look at yourself.

You may fear taking risks for several reasons: low self-esteem, lack of self-confidence, a history of repeated failure or disappointment. This roadblock is a tough one. To overcome it, you must take the time for an attitude adjustment. Think positively about making changes. Use your goal-setting skills. As we have mentioned, you might find it easier to set many, smaller short-term goals that will be easier to achieve and will boost your esteem.

Most people have one or more of these roadblocks. They stand in your way and keep you from reaching your goals. So take some time now to review thoroughly each of your roadblocks and come up with a plan of action to overcome them.

Goal-Tending

You've identified your roadblocks and their solutions. It's now time to write down each step you're going to take to reach your goals.

Creating this action plan is like drawing a ladder, with each step as a rung you must climb. Call it your "Goal Ladder." To identify your ladder's steps, start at your long-range goal and work backwards. Here's an example:

	DATE ACCOMPLISHED	GOAL	
Last date → at top	Nov. 18	Complete a 5 kilometer (3.1 mile) fun walk	← Final goal
	Nov. 12–18	Walk at least four times a week; walk at least 3 miles for two or more of the walks; walk at least 2½ miles for one or two of the walks.	
	Nov. 11	Do a practice five-kilometer walk	
	Oct. 28–Nov. 11	Walk at least four times a week; walk at least 2½ miles for two or more of the walks; walk at least 3 miles for one or two of the walks.	
	Oct. 14–27	Walk at least four days a week for 2 to 2½ miles each time. Send in registration for scheduled fun walk.	
	Sept. 16–Oct. 13	Walk at least four days a week for 1½ to 2 miles each time.	
Earliest date → on bottom	Sept. 1–16	Buy a new pair of walking shoes.	← First goal

YOUR GOAL LADDER

Use the Goal Ladder below to help you plan your action steps. Write your long-term goal on the top rung. On the rung below it, write the action step that must occur just before you reach your long-term goal. On the next rung down, write the action step that goes before the one above it. And so forth. Remember to make each action step realistic and specific. Your Goal Ladder can be as long or short as necessary to reach your goal. Put a completion date beside each action step.

DATE	GOAL

If this Goal Ladder works for you, develop several ladders, one for each short-range goal. This will help you break the effort down into "bite-size" pieces.

Reviewing Your Goals

A good way to see if you're staying on track is to review your Goal Ladder frequently. Remind yourself to do this by incorporating review times into your Goal Ladder as well as your completion date. These review times will help you take corrective action. They will also motivate you to try harder. Why? Because your progress will give you deep satisfaction and a great sense of accomplishment. And as you know, success is a great motivator!

CHAPTER

6

Get Set!

Walking has one big advantage over other types of exercise: *It requires little or no equipment.* All you really need is a comfortable pair of shoes. As for clothing, anything that's lightweight and feels good will do nicely. Plus, you can walk just about anywhere, just about anytime. So let's take a minute to learn how to choose walking shoes, socks, and workout clothes that are right for you.

Finding the Right Shoes

Technically speaking, you can walk in just about any shoe: high-heeled pumps, house slippers, flip-flops. But when you walk for health and fitness, you will want to leave these styles at home. Instead, look for comfortable shoes that support your feet. Think about it: For each mile you walk, your feet hit the ground between 1,500 and 2,000 times! So it pays to choose the right shoes. If your feet hurt, your fitness plans will go downhill fast.

The good news is that you have a lot to choose from. Most athletic sportswear companies have designed complete lines of shoes specifically for walking. Should you buy a "walking" shoe? Well, yes and no.

If you plan to do most of your walking in short bouts throughout the day (as lifestyle activities), the answer is no. Why? Because you'll quickly get tired of changing your shoes every time you go for a 5-minute walk. Instead, be sure the shoes you wear every day are comfortable.

Unfortunately, comfort and fashion don't always mix. You'll surely lose the desire to walk if you wear two-inch heels or classic wingtips. When your feet cramp and burn and you're in agony by noon, you'll say, "No way!" But don't worry. Several manufacturers have designed men's and women's shoes that combine the cushioning, support, and flexibility of athletic shoes with the style of fashion shoes. You can save yourself and your feet a lot of grief by checking into these hybrid shoes.

On the other hand, if you plan to walk for long stretches at a time or at a vigorous pace, an athletic-type walking shoe will probably work best. And while running shoes, tennis shoes, or aerobics shoes will certainly work, walking shoes are specially designed for the unique forces of the walking motion. Here's why:

☐ It's true that walking is a low-impact exercise, but you still hit the ground with a force of about one and one-half times your body weight. (Runners hit the ground with a force at least three times their body weight.) Your heel hits first and with the most force. Your weight then gradually transfers forward in a rolling motion through your arch and into the ball of your foot until you push off with your toes. Walking shoes are specially designed with a sole that's curved from heel to toe (like a rocker on a rocking chair) to help transfer your weight along the length of your foot.

☐ The flexible design of most walking shoes allows for an easy heel-to-toe rocking motion.

☐ Walking shoes have special cushioning to absorb shock throughout the sole, especially in the heel.

☐ In the back part of the shoe, special leather reinforcement adds stability to the heel. This is known as the heel counter.

☐ Walking shoes weigh about the same as most running shoes, but they are often lighter than aerobic shoes, cross-training shoes, and basketball shoes. When you're walking, a few extra ounces on each foot can really add up.

Did You Know?

Americans buy more walking shoes than any other sporting shoes. In fact, we buy over 46 million pairs of walking shoes per year. That adds up to over $1.8 billion in sales!

TO BUY OR NOT TO BUY

You're probably thinking that your old sneakers will fit the bill. But watch out. If they've been sitting in the back of your closet for the last four years, don't count on it. It's possible that your feet have changed shape slightly. Foot width and sometimes length increase slightly as we age. If you're going to walk a lot, that old pair of sneaks may cause you pain.

Sometimes a friend or family member wants to do you a favor by offering their old walking shoes. Even if you're exactly the same shoe size, your feet and the forces on your muscles and bones are as unique to you as your fingerprint. Wearing someone else's shoes can alter those forces and result in major discomfort and, possibly, injury.

 Tony decided to start walking early in the mornings before work to reduce his blood pressure level. He didn't think it was necessary to buy a new pair of shoes, since he knew his college-age son had the same size feet and a closet full of old sneakers.

After walking five days a week for three weeks, Tony started to feel a nagging ache in his right hip. He didn't think much about it until several weeks later, when the pain started to feel like a knife stab. He went to an orthopedic specialist who prescribed rest, pain killers, and physical therapy. It was the physical therapist who figured out that Tony was walking in used shoes.

Finally, after over $550 in medical expenses, Tony was convinced that a $60 investment in a new pair of shoes would have been worth the price.

If you need to buy new shoes for either a lifestyle or traditional type of walking program, heed the following for a good fit.

Shoe Buying Checklist

☐ Shop for shoes late in the day. Your feet are biggest in the late afternoon and evening after you've been walking around awhile.

☐ Use the type of socks that you will normally be wearing when walking (see 62–63 for suggestions).

☐ Check the insole (the inner padding of the shoe). If you wear orthotic devices, you will need to be able to remove the insole. A removable insole is also nice for easy cleaning and airing.

☐ Make sure the front of the shoe is wide so that your toes can spread easily as you roll off the front of your foot.

☐ The tip of your longest toe should not be any closer to the end of the shoe than about the width of a thumbnail. Have the salesperson or a friend test the length while you're standing squarely on both feet.

☐ After lacing, make sure the rows of lace holes on either side of the shoe are at least one inch apart. If they're too close, you don't have much room for adjustment. If they're more than a couple of inches apart, the shoe may be too tight.

☐ Stand on your tiptoes to make sure that your heel doesn't come out of the heel of the shoe.

☐ Walk briskly around the store to check for comfort and cushioning. Try to walk on a hard surface instead of soft carpet. Make sure the shoe bends easily under the ball of your foot. Be on the alert for tightness and rubbing, especially around the ankle or by your little toe. Notice how your arch feels. Make sure the shoe's arch support matches up with your foot's arch. You don't want the arch support to be too far forward or behind your arch. Also, you should just slightly feel the shoe's arch on the bottom of your foot. It should not be a constant, noticeable pressure on the arch of your foot.

☐ If you find a pair of shoes that really fits well after you have worn it at home awhile, consider going back and buying another pair or two of the same style. Shoe manufacturers regularly discontinue shoe lines to make room for newer models. Save the extra pair or two for future use, or rotate them with the pair currently in use.

You need new shoes if:

☐ The tread pattern is worn smooth.

☐ The tread becomes overly worn either on the inside or outside at the heel.

☐ The shoes don't feel as cushiony as when you first bought them.

☐ You start to develop pains in your hips, knees, or shins.

LACING TECHNIQUES

You may think that there's just one way to tie your shoes—the way you learned to do it at age three. Not true. There are several variations on the standard crisscross lacing technique. These different techniques boost your comfort level and prevent injuries.

If You Have:	*Try This Lacing Method:*
Loose heel or heel blisters	Technique #1
Narrow feet	Technique #1 or #2
Wide feet	Technique #3
High arches or pain on top of foot	Technique #4

Technique #1. Lace your shoe as you normally would through the second-to-the-last eyelet. Lace directly to the last eyelet on the same side. Then cross over to the opposite side and through the loop created there. This technique will help draw the heel tighter around your foot.

Technique #2. This method only works with shoes that have eyelet holes that are punched at variable widths on each side of the shoe's centerline (the middle of the tongue). Lace the eyelets that are farthest away from the centerline to draw the upper part of the shoe more tightly around your foot.

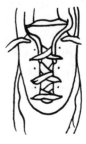

Technique #3. Again, this method works only on shoes with variable-width eyelets. Only lace the eyelets that are closest to the center-line. This will loosen the upper part of the shoe slightly.

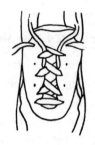

Technique #4. This method helps distribute the lace pressure more evenly because the laces don't crisscross over the top of the foot. With the toe of the shoe facing you, thread the laces downward (toward the tongue) through the first pair of eyelets (closest to the toe). Take the left lace and thread it out the third eyelet from the bottom on the left side. Thread the right lace out the second eyelet on the right

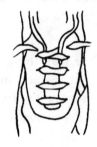

and then cross over and push the lace downward through the second eyelet on the left. Take the lace coming out of the third eyelet on the left and cross it over to the right side. Thread it downward through the third eyelet on the right side. Continue in this fashion until you get to the next-to-the-last eyelet on each side. Pull the laces through, cross over as with normal lacing, and insert the laces upward through the last eyelet on each side.

Sock It to Me

Big Tip Number One: Always wear socks when you walk. Socks help absorb sweat. They also cushion and prevent friction against your bare foot. "Fine," you say, "I have a drawer full of socks. No problem." Wait a minute. Just any sock won't do. Here's why:

- ☐ Dress socks, nylons, and pantyhose are too thin to prevent friction on a walk of any real length.
- ☐ Tube socks are just that—tubes of knitted fabric with an end sewn shut. They tend to bunch in the heel and toes, which can

hinder circulation and cause blisters. They also tend to ride high on the calf which can be uncomfortable, especially in hot weather.

☐ If your socks are threadbare or have holes, you may get blisters.

So, for walking comfort and blister prevention:

☐ Choose socks that fit without bunching anywhere. Be careful not to get them too small. That will put too much pressure on the ends of your toes.

☐ Since your feet will sweat, you will want a sock that's mostly acrylic to wick away moisture from the surface of your skin. All cotton socks tend to hold moisture at your feet and bunch when wet, which can cause blisters to form. Experiment with different varieties to find the style that works best for you.

☐ As for thickness, that's up to you. Just be sure to wear the same-weight socks you used when you first tried on your shoes. Otherwise, your shoes may feel too sloppy or tight.

Dressing for the Occasion

When it comes to walking, think "loose-fitting and lightweight." If you're following a lifestyle walking program, be sure that your day-to-day wardrobe is as comfortable as possible. That doesn't mean you have to wear a sweatsuit to work. On the other hand, if you're a woman, avoid wearing very short, tight skirts on the days you plan to do a lot of walking. If you're a man, shed that suit coat and loosen your tie while walking. And every walker should wear fabrics that breathe, such as cotton.

If you plan to follow a more traditional walking program, the "comfortable and lightweight" rules still apply. Aim for loose-fitting clothes that won't bind or constrict while you're bending, stretching, and walking. Don't wear anything that will restrict your breathing in any way.

If you're walking indoors, a single lightweight layer should be enough. But to prevent getting chilled, be sure to have a jacket or sweatshirt handy to put on afterwards.

If you're walking outdoors, be ready for all conditions. If the weather's warm, lightweight cotton clothing is your best bet. Unlike most other fabrics, cotton absorbs your perspiration and holds it close to your body. Your movement and any breeze slowly evaporates the moisture, which will help cool you. Other ways to stay cool are to wear shorts, tank tops, and T-shirts. On sunny days, use light-colored clothing to reflect some of the sun's rays. Cover your head, wear sunglasses, and, of course, use a waterproof sunscreen of at least SPF 15.

As the weather gets cooler, you can add layers, including a sweatshirt, windbreaker, gloves, and hat. The Boy Scout motto, "Be Prepared," is a good rule to apply to your walking program. If you're prepared, bad weather conditions shouldn't be a reason to fall off the walking "wagon."

Fill 'er Up!

How far do you think your car would go in hot weather with an empty radiator? Yeah, about as far as *you* would.

Drinking water is essential to life. It's even more important when you're physically active, especially in warm weather. Here's how it works: Each time you breathe out, you lose some moisture from your lungs. When you're walking briskly, your breathing rate increases and so does your water loss through respiration.

Also, you may sweat when you walk. That's your body's way of naturally cooling itself. As the sweat on your skin evaporates, it cools the skin's surface. The blood running through the tiny vessels in your skin releases some of its excess heat through the cooler skin surface. On windy days you may not notice that you're sweating because the wind dries any sweat immediately. But you're still losing fluid. So always rehydrate, whether you think you're sweating or not.

In fact, you can lose a great deal of water as you build up your walking program, especially in hot weather. Your game plan: Drink plenty of water before and after walking. This will greatly reduce your risk of overheating or heat exhaustion.

Hydration Tips

- Regardless of the type of walking program you're doing, drink plenty of water throughout the day. Don't count caffeinated or alcoholic beverages. They contain substances that actually cause your system to lose water.
- If you are following a traditional walking program, get in the habit of drinking six to eight ounces of water right before and right after you walk.

- If you're going for a long or fast walk in hot, humid weather, weigh yourself before you walk and immediately afterwards. The difference in weight is due to water loss (not fat loss!). You must replace the lost water by drinking two cups (sixteen ounces) of water for every pound lost. For example, if you lost two pounds, you need to drink four cups, or thirty-two ounces. The sooner you rehydrate yourself, the more quickly you'll recover.
- Water is all you need. Special sports drinks provide a lot of calories and little else. If one of your goals is to lose weight, you'll be defeating your purpose. If you want something sweet to drink, try orange or cranberry juice mixed with an equal amount of water.
- If you're going for a long walk, make sure there's a way to get some water along the way, or take water along with you. Most sports stores offer handy belts with pouches that will easily hold a water bottle.
- Don't rely on feeling thirsty to tell you when to drink. Your internal thirst mechanism sometimes lags behind your body's actual needs, especially when you're sweating a lot. And as you get older, your thirst mechanism is simply not as accurate as when you were younger. Try to drink water at 15- to 20-minute intervals during your walk.

The last of the loose ends has been tied. You're ready to walk! The next chapter will help you take the first steps.

CHAPTER

7

Let's Go for a Walk!

Now you're ready for a fun and invigorating walk. Before you take off, consider a few pointers that can help make your walk safe, effective, and enjoyable.

Begin With a Warm-Up

While it's tempting to just start out cold, do your muscles a favor and warm them up first. Warm muscles are less likely to be pulled or injured. Plus, it gives you time to get your heart rate up a bit before the big event. Aim for 5 minutes of slow walking or other warm-up exercises before setting out, especially if you plan to walk rapidly or if the weather is cold. If you're following a traditional exercise plan, try reaching your target heart rate by the end of your warm-up period.

There are many benefits of a warm-up before you exercise:

☐ It stimulates circulation and increases your heart rate.
☐ It increases body (and muscle) temperature.
☐ It prevents soreness and injury.
☐ It heightens your awareness of how your body feels.

STRETCHING EXERCISES

The following stretching exercises are great for walkers. If your muscles are tight, you can do them as a warm-up before walking.

They'll help you loosen up and relax before you walk. They can also be used as you cool down after your walk. One advantage of stretching at the end of your walk is that your muscles are well warmed and less likely to be strained. (For more cool-down stretching exercises, see page 77–79.)

These stretches can be done anytime. If taken slowly, they can even be done while watching television at home, while working at the office, or while waiting at the bus stop. Many people get tense neck and shoulder muscles, especially at work. The neck stretches and shoulder circles are great for relieving the tension in these muscles. In fact, all of these stretches are a good way to help you loosen up—wherever you are. They are also a great way to relieve tension any time you feel stressed.

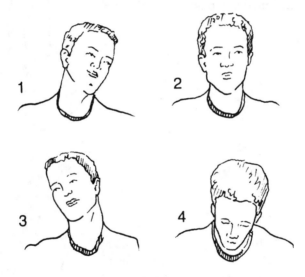

Neck Stretches. While sitting or standing with your head in its normal upright position, slowly tilt your head to the left until you feel tightness on the right side of your neck (1). Hold for 10 to 15 seconds, then return your head to the upright position (2). Repeat to the right side (3), and then toward the front (4). Always return to the upright position before moving on. **Do not tilt your head back.**

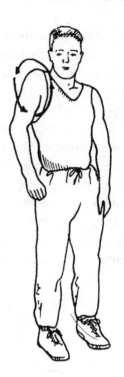

Shoulder Circles. While sitting or standing, rotate your shoulders in the backward direction. Be sure to go through the full range of motion. Because most people have a slight case of rounded shoulders due to desk work, housework, or other tasks, forward shoulder circles aren't necessary. Older people have a fairly limited range of motion and need to be careful when doing this stretch. Just do what you can, but don't push beyond your limits.

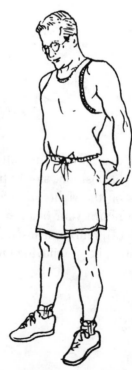

Chest Stretch. Stand and clasp your hands behind your back and stretch your chest muscles by pulling your shoulder blades together. Also, perform the chest stretch while bending forward at the waist and lifting your clasped hands away from your lower back toward the ceiling.

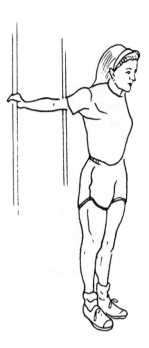

Chest Pull. Stand facing a door frame. Place your hands on the frame at shoulder level and walk through the doorway until you feel a slight tension in your chest muscles.

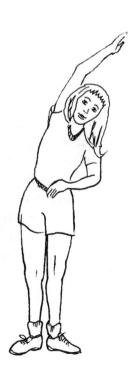

Side Bends. Stand with your feet shoulder-width apart. Extend one arm overhead and place the hand of the other arm on your hip. Bend to the side opposite the lifted arm. Extend the other arm overhead and repeat the bend to the opposite side. Older people need to be careful with this stretch. Bend only as far as you can.

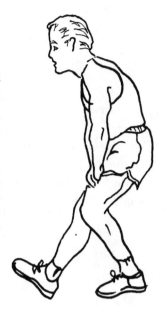

Hamstring Stretches. Stand with your feet shoulder-width apart and extend the right foot in front of the left and parallel to it. Bend your left leg about halfway, and keep your right leg straight with the foot flexed. Flex your right foot as much as possible to achieve the maximum stretch in the back of your right thigh. Keep your weight centered between your feet. Place both hands on your left thigh for upper body support. Repeat with opposite leg.

Calf Stretches. Stand with your feet together and parallel. Step with one foot forward so that your feet are approximately one to two feet apart. Gently shift your weight onto your front leg, being sure to keep your back straight and your back toes directed forward. Keep both heels on the floor. You can rest your hands on your front leg for stability.

As you do these stretches, remember:

☐ Stretch slowly and smoothly. Don't bounce in an attempt to increase the stretch.

☐ Stretch only as far as it's comfortable. Never stretch to the point of pain.

☐ Be sure that support is nearby (a wall, a tree, another person) before doing a stretch that requires balance.

☐ Breathe while stretching. Inhale before the stretch and exhale during the stretch.

☐ Hold each stretch for 10 to 20 seconds. Do each stretch three to five times.

If you're taking the lifestyle approach to exercise, it's still a good idea to warm up gradually as you begin. Suppose you're planning to walk 10 minutes to the deli down the street for lunch. Start off at an easy pace. If your muscles are tight, take a few seconds to do some gentle stretches. For example, if you plan to tackle several flights of stairs, start with calf stretches.

Sitting Pretty, Standing Straight

Although it sounds like something your mother would say, proper posture *is* important. No kidding. Oh, sure, it helps you look good and project a positive self-image. But what it also does is help your body achieve balance. It keeps your body aligned so that it moves more efficiently with minimum strain and effort. It will also cut down on the aches and pains that can result if your body is not aligned.

In the illustration on page 72, notice that the figure on the right is standing with good posture. The ear lobe, tip of the shoulder, middle of the hips, back of the kneecap, and front of the anklebone are in a verticle line. The figure on the left is using poor posture. If you were to connect the body segments in that figure, you would have a broken line.

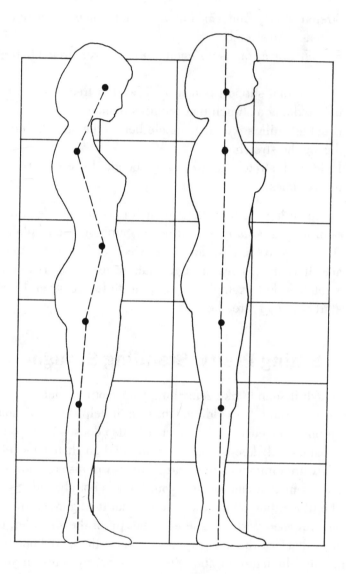

Standing Posture

The Standing Posture Checklist

Stand in front of a mirror to check your posture, or ask a friend to help you.

____ Are you standing as tall as possible without straining?

____ Is your head erect with your neck centered between your shoulders?

____ Is the back of your head in line with the back of your heels and centered over your spine?

____ Are your shoulders straight and level, but not tense?

____ Do your shoulders line up with your hips, knees, and ankles?

____ Are your shoulder blades wide apart and pressed down?

____ Are your arms relaxed and hanging loosely by your sides?

____ Is your chest moderately elevated?

____ Are your abdominal muscles held firm and tight?

____ Are your buttocks tilted down and under, tilting your pelvis upward in front?

____ Is your pelvis aligned directly under your torso?

____ Is your pelvis level and centered squarely above your feet?

____ Are your knees straight without being stiff, locked, or extended too far backwards?

____ Are your knees directly under your hip joints?

____ Is your body weight centered between the heels and balls of both feet in front of your ankles?

____ Are your feet parallel and pointed forward or slightly outward?

IF YOU ARE SLOUCHING . . . HERE'S HELP

Okay, so you have poor posture. That may be because of weak or imbalanced muscles. These muscles can—and should—be corrected before they cause permanent structural abnormalities.

A common posture problem for walkers is swayback. That's when your spine curves too much at the lower back. It often results in low-back pain. Fortunately, you can improve or correct swayback by strengthening the lower abdominal muscles and increasing the flexibility of the lower back muscles. Weak abdominal muscles allow your pelvis to tilt forward and increase the curve of your lower back. So, too, do inflexible hamstrings and lower back muscles. Good muscle tone in the buttocks is important too, since the buttocks help to lift the pelvis upward.

The following exercises can help to improve your posture and reduce low-back pain. Perform the floor exercises on a comfortable surface. A carpeted floor or an exercise mat is best. Do them in a controlled, rhythmic manner. If you feel any discomfort or pain, **stop exercising immediately.**

Posture Exercises

Position: Lie on your back with your knees bent and your feet flat on the floor.

- Place the palms of your hands on your thighs. Lift your shoulders off the floor and slide your fingers up toward your knees. The movement will be small, only a few inches. Return to the starting position and repeat. Do as many repetitions as you can, working up to 25.
- Place your arms by your sides with your palms down. Contract your abdominal muscles and buttocks at the same time so that your back is flattened against the floor. Hold the contraction for 6 seconds, relax, and repeat the movement 10 to 20 times.
- Place your arms by your sides. Contract your abdominals and flatten your back against the floor. Raise your head while bringing both knees to your chest. Clasp both hands around your knees. Pull tightly and hold for 6 seconds. Relax and return to the floor. Repeat the movement 10 to 20 times.
- Raise your head and bring one knee as close to your chest as possible. Keep your other leg relaxed. Return your raised leg to the floor and lower your head. Repeat with your other leg. Perform 5 of these movements on each side, working up to 10 repetitions.

MINI-TEST: WATCH YOURSELF WALK

The next time you see your reflection in a store window while walking, pay attention to your posture and gait. As you walk, you'll make adjustments in your posture to ensure stability and balance. Here are the basic elements of a good walking gait:

☐ Begin with an erect standing posture and then shift your body weight forward slightly from your ankles.

☐ Start your leg swing at the hip and move forward with a minimum of movement to the side.

☐ Point your feet straight ahead and place them just to the left and right of an imaginary center line. Most people walk with about three inches between their feet.

☐ Push off each step from your toes.

☐ Swing your arms freely and naturally, but keep your shoulders level and parallel, not raised.

☐ Move your arms in opposition to your legs to keep your body facing forward.

☐ Ease your body weight onto your supporting foot to minimize impact. Strike your heel first and then the ball of your foot.

☐ Keep your stride moderate in length, allowing your knees to be slightly flexed as your legs swing forward and your feet strike the ground.

RELIEF FROM LOW-BACK PAIN

If you suffer from low-back pain, here are some suggestions that can help. Don't let back pain become a reason for not walking!

☐ Avoid standing in one position for an extended period of time. When you do that, it becomes difficult to keep your hips from sagging forward, and this will strain your lower back.

☐ Always bend your knees when leaning forward, lifting, or lowering objects.

☐ Avoid carrying objects above elbow level.

☐ If you sleep on your stomach, place a pillow under your abdomen for support.

☐ If you sleep on your side, place a pillow between your legs to keep your body properly aligned.

☐ When lying on your back, place a pillow under the bend of your knees so that your back does not over-flex.

☐ When sitting, keep your thighs parallel to the floor or slightly higher than your hips.

☐ When driving, adjust the seat position so that you can reach the pedals without strain.

☐ Avoid any position that places your head and neck forward while thrusting your chin upward.

Don't Forget to Breathe

It sounds silly, but breathing is basic to life—and walking. When you walk at a brisk pace, your rate of breathing and your heart rate increase. It's important to breathe deeply and evenly through your nose *and* mouth as you walk. This technique allows you to take in the maximum amount of air.

Remember the Talk Test? If you're talking comfortably while walking briskly, you're right on target. If you're breathing so hard that you can't talk, you're probably walking too fast. As your fitness level improves, you'll be able to walk faster without being out of breath.

BREATHING EASIER

If you have allergies, asthma, or other respiratory problems, don't worry. Just be sure to check with your doctor before beginning an exercise program. He or she may prescribe an inhaler for you to use before you work out. It may help you breathe easier. There are nasal inhalers for hay fever and sinus allergies, as well as oral inhalers for asthma. Your doctor will tell you how and when to use them. Once you establish an activity program, your lung capacity should increase. This will let you breathe more deeply and comfortably. Regular exercise can actually be therapeutic for allergy and asthma sufferers.

LIFE AND BREATH

If you're a smoker, walking for exercise may be difficult. Smoking slows you down, but you, too, can make progress. Think about using walking to help you break the cigarette habit. Walking will:

- ☐ help relieve the symptoms of nicotine withdrawal
- ☐ give you something to do to get your mind off of smoking
- ☐ burn extra calories to help control your weight

Many smokers who've started a walking program report that they've finally been able to give up cigarettes for good.

WORKING OUT AT THE RIGHT PACE

If you're going the traditional exercise route, find out if you're working out at the right pace by monitoring your heart rate. Adjust your pace to stay within your target heart rate zone. It's a good idea to take your pulse at several points throughout your walk, especially:

- ☐ before your walk (resting heart rate)
- ☐ after your warm-up phase
- ☐ every 4 to 5 minutes while walking (target heart rate)
- ☐ after your cool-down phase

Rating your perceived exertion can also help you monitor the intensity of your workout. You can use it with either the traditional or a lifestyle approach to exercise. The Talk Test works well for gauging lifestyle walking programs. Review pages 44–45 for recommendations about intensity levels that are appropriate for your current fitness.

Cooling Down Is Really Cool

After your workout, start to slow down gradually. Keep walking, but slow your pace to a stroll. This cool-down period:

- ☐ allows your heart rate and breathing rate to return to normal gradually
- ☐ prevents dizziness by avoiding the pooling of blood in your legs
- ☐ helps regulate your body temperature

Checking your heart rate at the end of your cool-down is an excellent way to evaluate your workout and fitness level. After about 5 minutes of cool-down, your heart rate should be below 120 if you're younger than age 50 and below 110 if you're over age 50. If your heart rate is not at or below these levels, rest for 5 more minutes and then check your heart rate again. If your heart rate is still not at or below these levels, your workout was too strenuous. Rest for 5 minutes more and check your heart rate once more. If your heart rate was still not at or below the levels listed, check with your doctor. Also be sure to check with your doctor if at any time during the workout or after you feel any of the symptoms listed on page 85.

COOL-DOWN STRETCHES

Your cool-down phase is an ideal time to do stretching exercises because your muscles are warm and your joints are more flexible. (For more stretching exercises, see pages 66–70.) The cool-down phase is also a good time to add a few relaxation techniques to help with stress management.

Thigh Stretches. Stand facing a wall. Place your right hand against the wall at shoulder level for balance. Bend your left leg at the knee. Using your left hand, grasp the top of your left foot behind you. Gently pull your heel toward your buttocks. Repeat for the other side.

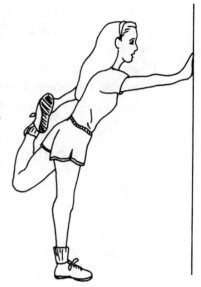

Alternate Thigh Stretches. Lie on your left side with your head resting in the palm of your left hand. Hold the top of your right foot between the toes and ankle joint with your right hand. Gently pull the right heel toward the right buttock. Turn over and re-peat for the other side.

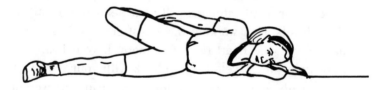

Inner Thigh Stretch. Sit on the floor. Place the soles of your feet together with your knees pointed outward. Pull your heels in as close to the buttocks as possible. Slowly press the knees down towards the floor as you lean forward from the hips.

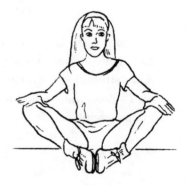

Calf Stretches. Stand with your feet together and parallel. Step forward with one foot so that your feet are approximately one to two feet apart. Gently shift your weight onto your front leg, being sure to keep your back straight and your back toes directed forward. Keep both heels on the floor. You can rest your hands on your front leg for stability.

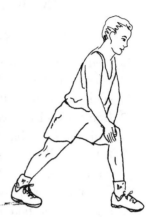

How to Keep From Getting Injured

The risk of an exercise-related injury while walking is very small. Still, injuries *can* occur. The most common ones for walkers are caused by overuse. Don't try to do too much too soon, or walk too fast for too long.

The Four S's of Walking Safety

☐ Shoes—Get a good pair of shoes, ideally one specifically designed for walking.

☐ Stretch—Stretch the muscles and tendons that you use in walking as part of your cool-down or warm-up, or at any other available time.

☐ Surface—Walk on a resilient surface if possible. A grassy or smooth dirt surface is excellent. If you must walk on a very hard surface, good walking shoes are even more important. Avoid rough, uneven surfaces.

☐ Style—The faster you walk, the more you must change your style. Adjust your posture by leaning forward *slightly* and bending and pumping your arms as you quicken your pace.

COMMON SENSE GUIDELINES

Using common sense will help make your walking program safe.

☐ Don't exercise strenuously for at least two hours after a meal.

☐ Do only mild, low-intensity exercise if you have a minor illness such as a cold or flu.

☐ Don't exercise if you have a fever, and don't resume exercise until the fever has been gone for at least twenty-four hours.

☐ After an illness, cut back your time and intensity of exercise for a while.

☐ Pay attention to your body. If you notice that a blister is forming, stop and take care of what's causing it immediately.

☐ Expect some mild soreness when you're first starting to be more active or after you increase your pace or intensity. Delayed soreness occurs for a day or two after a change in your activity and disappears as your body makes adjustments. Massage can help relax sore muscles.

Exercising Caution: Knowing the Warning Signs of Heart Attack

If you're physically active, you need to know the warning signs that may indicate a heart attack. *Stop exercising immediately if any of these symptoms occur, and see your doctor before resuming exercise:*

☐ uncomfortable pressure, fullness, squeezing, or pain in the center of the chest lasting more than a few minutes

☐ pain spreading to the shoulders, neck, or arms

☐ chest discomfort with lightheadedness, fainting, sweating, nausea, or shortness of breath

---

Walking in the Great Outdoors

Your community probably has many wonderful places for you to walk outdoors. The most convenient place may be right outside your back door. Many neighborhoods have shady trees and lovely gardens. You've probably seen them as you whizzed by in your car. These sights are even more enjoyable when you walk by them.

Another nice thing about walking in your neighborhood is that it gives you an opportunity to meet your neighbors. You can even ask them to join you on your walk. Invite them over for juice and coffee afterward.

Your community probably has many places you can walk. Local parks and recreation centers often have walking tracks. Some schools have outdoor tracks that can be used for walking. Even many hospitals and businesses have created mini walking paths.

One way to find places to walk in your community is to call a local walking club. You can probably find their address or phone number in your local newspaper or on the bulletin board at your local community center. If you don't find a listing, ask the recreation director at the community center. He or she can probably help you find a walking club or help get one started.

Almost all communities have some wonderful places to walk and enjoy the great outdoors. Just see which ones suit you the best.

FINDING A SAFE PLACE TO WALK

Most people enjoy walking outdoors, but sometimes that isn't possible because of potential hazards. It's not always sunny days and singing birds. Sometimes there's darkness, cold, traffic, fierce dogs, heatstroke, and other barriers you need to know how to handle. Here are a few common hazards and ideas to help you deal with them.

Dogs. Don't run from a dog. But don't stare him down, scream, or make advances toward him. Instead, walk briskly to the other side of the street. Choose a different route in the future.

Traffic. Always walk facing the oncoming traffic. Stay on sidewalks, if possible. Cross streets only at intersections and after looking both ways. Watch out for drivers who are turning on red. Don't wear earphones that would keep you from hearing the sounds associated with traffic. Air pollution in heavy traffic areas can also be a problem, so avoid it if you can.

Darkness. If you must walk when it's dark, wear light-colored or reflective clothing. Many sports stores sell reflective vests, arm bands, and leg bands. If possible, carry a lightweight flashlight. Avoid uneven surfaces that might cause you to trip or stumble.

Personal Safety. Walk with a partner, if possible. Carry a whistle or personal safety alarm. Leave valuables (jewelry, money, etc.) at home. Avoid areas that seem risky. Carry identification and a small amount of money in a fanny pack.

Air Pollution. Avoid walking outside if the air quality is poor, especially during ozone alerts. If you live or work in an area where traffic or industrial pollution is a problem, look for a place to walk with clean indoor air, such as a shopping mall that doesn't allow smoking on the premises. Also, avoid areas with heavy pollen, mold, and spores. You can reduce your exposure to environmental hazards by walking outdoors early in the morning, late in the evening, and on weekends.

High Altitude. Don't be caught off-guard if you are planning to walk or hike at high altitudes. In higher elevations, the barometric pressure decreases and the air becomes thinner. With each breath, there is less oxygen to breathe, so you become fatigued more easily. Your body adjusts to high altitudes by increasing its production of red blood cells so that more oxygen can be delivered to your muscles. No two people adjust to increases in altitude exactly the same way, even if they're extremely fit.

Symptoms of mountain sickness may include shortness of breath, headaches, dizziness, and nausea. In most people, minor symptoms will disappear within twenty-four to forty-eight hours. It may take several weeks to adjust completely. If your symptoms are severe, it's advisable to descend to lower altitudes as soon as possible.

To help prevent mountain sickness or minimize its symptoms, get enough rest and sleep, drink lots of water, and avoid alcohol for the first couple of days. Avoid smoking. Poor health, particularly cardiovascular and pulmonary disease, can contribute to problems at altitudes over 5,000 feet. If you have medical concerns, talk with your doctor before walking or hiking at high altitudes.

LETTING THE WEATHER CHOOSE YOUR CLOTHES

When you start your walking program, you'll want to dress for success. That means not wearing clothes that are uncomfortable or too cold in the winter or hot in the summer.

COLD WEATHER

The major dangers of walking in extremely cold weather are frostbite and hypothermia. Symptoms of frostbite include numbness and white discoloration of the skin, especially on your hands, ears, toes, and face. Hypothermia—when your body temperature drops rapidly to dangerous levels—is mostly a risk when you're out in very cold weather for many hours, especially if you're wet or not moving around enough to stay warm.

Both frostbite and hypothermia can be avoided by a taking a few precautions:

- ☐ Warm up and stretch before going outdoors when it's cold.
- ☐ Pay careful attention to the windchill factor, and dress accordingly.
- ☐ In extreme cold or during high windchill, wear a hat, gloves, and thick socks. Wrap a scarf around the head, neck, and face. Wear sunglasses and sunscreen.
- ☐ Keep your head covered at all times.
- ☐ Dress in layers. It's better to wear too much than not enough.
- ☐ Wear a windbreaker with a front zipper for the outer layer.
- ☐ Remove or open outer layers before sweating makes under layers wet.
- ☐ If you get chilled, put the other layer back on.
- ☐ If your clothing becomes wet for any reason, go indoors and change as soon as possible.
- ☐ Drink plenty of water. You can become dehydrated not only from sweating, but also by exhaling moist air.
- ☐ Keep moving to stay warm.

RAIN, RAIN GO AWAY

Rain is a reason many people give for missing their walks. But just like the mailman, you can't let rain keep you from your appointed duty. Have a back-up activity to do on rainy days. Or simply get out and enjoy the cool freshness of a gentle rain. Keep these things in mind:

- ☐ Wear a light waterproof slicker or jacket. Make sure it's not too tight and is made of a fabric that breathes. Ponchos work expecially well because they allow lots of freedom for arm movement, and air can circulate freely underneath.
- ☐ Wear a hat with a wide brim or a hood. It is hard to walk with an umbrella, especially if it's windy.

☐ Make sure your shoes have rubber soles and a good tread. They are less inclined to slip when wet.

☐ Watch out for leaves, grass, and mud in your path. They can be very slick.

☐ Dry your shoes thoroughly before using them again. One good way to dry walking shoes is to stuff them with paper towels or newspaper. They should be dry in about twenty-four hours. If not, replace the paper towels or newspaper and let them dry another twenty-four hours. This is why it is a good idea to have a second pair on hand.

☐ Acknowledge that you will probably get at least a little wet. Except for the wicked witch in *The Wizard of Oz*, a little water never hurt anyone. Besides, it is part of the fun of walking in the rain!

If it's raining too hard or if you don't want to walk in the rain, you don't have to give up your walk. Just look for a place with clean indoor air. Try your local mall, community center, or place of worship.

THE HOT-WEATHER MODE

The major dangers of extremely hot weather are dehydration, heat exhaustion, and heatstroke. These risks are especially grave if the humidity is above 70 percent. Heat and humidity interfere with the body's natural cooling process.

In hot weather, especially if it's humid, try to walk in the early morning or late evening. You may need to walk slower and for a shorter period. Wear light, loose clothing that allows air to get to your skin.

Know the symptoms of heat exhaustion and heatstroke. If any of these symptoms appear, take action immediately to cool down by dousing yourself with cold water. Seek medical attention if necessary. Heat exhaustion can progress quickly to heatstroke, a potentially fatal condition.

Wear very light, comfortable clothing, and when it's hot, walk in the early morning or late evening, if possible.

Symptoms of Heat Exhaustion

Stop walking immediately if you have any of these symptoms:

☐ Heavy sweating and cold, clammy skin
☐ Dizziness
☐ A rapid pulse
☐ Throbbing pressure in your head
☐ Chills
☐ Flushed appearance
☐ Nausea

Symptoms of Heatstroke

☐ Warm, dry skin with no sweating *or* heavy sweating and cold, clammy skin
☐ Low blood pressure
☐ Confusion and/or unconsciousness
☐ High fever
☐ A slow pulse
☐ Ashen or gray skin

HAVE WATER BOTTLE, WILL TRAVEL

If your walk is going to be longer than 30 to 45 minutes, carry a water bottle with you. Regardless of the weather, drink water before, during, and after walking. Don't depend on thirst to let you know you need to drink more water. That's not always a good indicator. See pages 64–65 for specific recommendations on how to stay safe by drinking plenty of water.

CHAPTER

Staying Motivated

What Are You Up To?

Are you up to starting—and sticking with—a regular walking plan? Great! Now you need the secret to staying on track for the long haul: *motivation.*

Almost everyone knows that success is a great motivator. In every aspect of our lives, small successes lead to bigger ones. So it's critical that you take the time to savor the taste of success at each of your walking milestones.

In this chapter, we'll offer a variety of techniques to help you enjoy your successes and stay on track. We'll also show you how to get back on track when inevitable lapses put you temporarily on the sidelines.

Tracking Your Success

Start by reviewing your goals. Where do you want to be in a week? A month? A year? There's only one way to make sure you'll get there, and that's to carefully track your progress every step of the way.

One excellent tracking tool is the Personal Data Record in Appendix III. If you consistently fill in this form, you'll see at a glance how your physical fitness, blood pressure, blood cholesterol, and body weight change over time. And that's important, because these conditions directly affect your heart. Sedentary living habits, high blood pressure, obesity, and a high blood cholesterol level are all risk factors for heart disease. But as you become more active through walking, you'll begin to see positive changes in some of these areas, and they'll be evident as you track your record.

When you fill out your Personal Data Record, use the "Other" category to keep track of other health-related variables. For example, you may want to record your body measurements (thigh, hip, waist, chest, and upper arm circumferences) to see how they change over time. Or you could record blood glucose or triglycerides levels. The suggested time intervals are just guidelines; feel free to adjust them as you see fit. The more often you take these measurements (for example, once a week), the less likely you are to see big improvements. Weekly health measurements may also be too costly. Remember: You don't have to assess every health factor at each interval. Simply set a regular schedule that works for you.

After a few assessments, your Personal Data Record might look something like this.

Interval	Date	One-Mile Fitness Test			Body Weight	Blood Pressure	Blood Cholesterol	Other
		Time (min.: sec.)	Heart Rate	Fitness Category				
Base-line	10/13	18:30	140	Low	157	128/84	218	Thigh = 25; Waist = 34; Chest = 38
One Month	11/15	17:05	140	Moderate	155	128/80	—	Thigh = 24; Waist = 34; Chest = 38
Six Months	4/20	16:05	130	High	148	122/78	205	Thigh = 23; Waist = 31; Chest = 36

Don't be discouraged if you fail to see dramatic changes at first. The rate of change varies greatly depending on the amount of walking you do. So if you only walk a little during each interval, you probably won't see a big change. Remember that other factors, such as your diet, also play a part. Diet can affect your weight, blood pressure, and cholesterol level. See Chapter 11 for more information on the role your diet plays.

KEEP A WALKING DIARY

Here's an easy way to find out if you're reaching your goal. Simply record what you accomplish each day in a daily walking diary or log. But don't just record times and distances, also use your log to record other elements of your walk, including how you feel about your day's efforts. With a regular log, you'll be able to spot patterns in your activities that may help or hinder your walking efforts.

 For nearly three years, May walked at least five days a week. In the beginning, she could barely walk around the block without getting winded, but she made steady progress, eventually able to walk two miles each time.

But one week, May noticed that she was struggling as she walked. She felt sluggish and tired even before she began. Her walking pace dropped significantly, and instead of feeling invigorated when she was finished, she felt exhausted. In fact, she was so frustrated, she wanted to quit.

Fortunately, May kept a walking log. One evening as she was entering her day's data, she decided to look back over the preceding weeks. She noticed that her walking times began to suffer when she switched from walking in the morning to walking after work. Since it was early summer, the evenings were getting extremely warm. May realized that she probably had not properly prepared herself for walking in the heat and humidity.

Knowing the reason for her difficulty, May immediately felt better. She cut back her distance to a mile and a half and slowed to a comfortable pace until she became accustomed to the heat. She also carried a water bottle with her to prevent dehydration. May's careful diary entries helped save her walking program.

___

We have included a diary in this book in Appendix I. It includes a sample diary that has been filled in and is followed by a blank diary for you to fill in. Use it to help you monitor your day-to-day walking. Take a moment now to look at it. You'll see that the log has:

☐ Two pages for each week, with a summary section for you to fill in at the end of the week.

☐ A place for you to record the date.

☐ Space on the Monday of each week for you to write your weekly goals and rewards.

☐ A place to record the specifics about your daily walking efforts (where you walk, the overall intensity of your walks, the time and distance of each walk, etc.). Notice that there's plenty of space for you to record information. You may not need all of it unless you are using the "lifestyle" approach to walking. At the end of each day, you can list the time and/or distance for the day and add it to your weekly total.

☐ Space for you to keep track of your other physical activities.

☐ A checklist in the summary to remind you that every workout needs to include warm-up, cool-down, and stretching phases.

☐ Several lines for you to record any other details about your walking program. You can describe how you felt, the temperature, what you thought about on your walk—anything!

LOGGING LOGISTICS

Here are some helpful tips for making your walking diary pay real dividends.

☐ *Carry the diary with you.* If it sits on a shelf at home, you're likely to forget to make regular entries.

☐ *Record your activity immediately* (with the exception of the "Comments" section). It's amazing how quickly you can forget important details. Add your thoughts and feelings later in the day when you've had time to ponder them.

☐ *Record something every day.* "Even if I don't walk at all?" you ask. Yes! *Especially* then. Describe the reasons why you didn't walk. For example, you needed to take some days as rest days. Or you were injured and couldn't walk for a while. Or maybe you just weren't motivated that day. Addressing exactly why you didn't walk may be enough to keep a simple lapse from becoming a more dangerous relapse.

☐ *Create your own diary.* To continue your log past the twelfth week, make copies of pages 144–167. Or design your own log—one that exactly meets your needs and interests.

☐ *Use it or lose it.* Remember, keeping a walking log is a powerful motivational tool, but it only works if you use it.

HOW FAR HAVE YOU WALKED?

Timing your walks is easy. All you need is a watch. But how can you learn how far you walk each day? If you're walking on a track, you can count laps. If you're walking in the neighborhood, you can drive the distance, clocking it on your car's odometer. Or you can estimate the distance covered by the time and intensity of your walk. How? Time yourself on a one-mile measured track. If you walk the mile in 15 minutes, you can get a feel for that pace. As you take your daily walk, try to match the pace you remember from your experience on the track. If you feel you're walking at the same pace as you did on the track, about 15 minutes per mile, and you walk for 45 minutes, then you probably walked about three miles.

But to know *exactly* how far you walk, get a pedometer, a handy gadget for calculating distance while walking or running. Sporting goods stores have many different types and styles. They range in price from about $15 to $50, depending on their features. They all operate on the same basic principle: You wear the pedometer on your waistband or belt, and a tiny pendulum inside the pedometer detects when you take a step with either foot.

Some pedometers simply record the number of steps you take. This is especially useful with a lifestyle walking program because it keeps you from having to write down all of your brief, two-minute walks. Simply wear this type of pedometer all day long to get an average number of steps per day. In subsequent weeks, try to increase the average number of steps by 5 to 10 percent.

Other models require that you code your stride length (see below) into the pedometer. It then multiplies the number of steps by the stride length to come up with the distance traveled. Because stride length can vary a lot throughout the day, this type of pedometer is best suited for a single long walk, when you generally use a consistent stride.

How to Measure Your Stride

To measure your stride length, mark two lines on the sidewalk 30 feet apart. Start walking about 20 feet away from the first mark and walk past the second mark a few steps (make sure that your stride lengths are the same as when you fitness walk). Count the number of steps you took between the two marks. Divide the distance you walked (30 feet) by the number of steps you took between the marks. For example, if you took 12 steps in the 30-foot distance, you divide 30 by 12 and get 2½. That means your stride length is 2½ feet. Your stride length will change as you become more physically fit, so be sure to check it periodically.

Some pedometers have "fancy" features, such as the ability to estimate the number of calories burned. It's a nice feature, but since the pedometer can't tell the intensity at which you are walking, the measurement is not very accurate. Keep this in mind when looking at some of the more expensive models.

CELEBRATING YOUR MILESTONES

In your daily log, you're going to achieve goals and pass milestones. They may be personal time or distance records, or the date of a significant event related to walking. Appendix IV provides a place where you can record these milestones. The following is an example of a "Walking Milestone" record.

Date	Milestone Description
6/23	Walked a mile without stopping for the first time!
7/4	Got the family to walk with me for 30 minutes before the big Fourth of July parade.
9/8	Walked two miles for the first time! I'm on my way!
9/30	I have walked fifty miles since I started!
10/23	Walked in my first five-kilometer fun run. What a blast!

Take time often to read through your list of achievements—they'll make you feel good about yourself and what you've accomplished.

Getting Your Just Desserts

Whatever you do, when you achieve a small goal, reward yourself!

Too often people fail to congratulate themselves properly with a tangible reward. Perhaps they don't feel they deserve it, or they have the feeling that "it's no big deal." But even the smallest accomplishment is a big deal if it puts you on the road to a healthy lifestyle, and rewards are super motivators. They give you something to look forward to and strive toward. They also make achieving your goals fun and enjoyable. For a reward to be motivating, it must be something you value. It also should be commensurate with the goal achieved. For example, giving yourself a compact disc player each day that you walk is not appropriate. But a compact disc player may be perfect when you reach your 1,000-mile goal.

Use the space below to list ways you can reward yourself. Organize your rewards by cost or value. Generally, you should use the more significant rewards for long-term goals or major milestone achievements. We've started you off with a few examples, but get creative. Come up with items that really matter to you.

Intangible Rewards	Tangible Rewards
➤ Relaxing bubble bath or hot shower	➤ Sports massage
➤ Call an old friend long-distance	➤ New sports watch
➤ _____	➤ Magazine subscription
➤ _____	➤ Weekend getaway
➤ _____	➤ _____
➤ _____	➤ _____
➤ _____	➤ _____
➤ _____	➤ _____
➤ _____	➤ _____
➤ _____	➤ _____
➤ _____	➤ _____
➤ _____	➤ _____

How often you reward yourself is up to you. Some people do best when they reward themselves every day. Others do better with weekly or monthly goals and rewards. You'll probably find that your preference as to the timing of your rewards will change as your walking program changes.

How to Have a One-Track Mind

No matter how clear your goals, how meticulous your records, and how motivating your rewards, you are going to have occasional difficulties. Illness, injury, family crises, job commitments, and other surprises may derail you from time to time. This is a natural part of making any change in your life. But it's important to recognize in advance that these setbacks will occur. Your goal? Keep them as temporary as possible and try to prevent them from happening again in the future.

These temporary setbacks are known as lapses. A relapse occurs when a lapse or series of lapses get strung out for several weeks and you end up back where you started.

AVOIDING THOSE PESKY LAPSES

You'll find that there are people, places, days, or other situations that put you at risk for abandoning your walking. And many are unique to you. It's important that you identify these high-risk situations and develop plans in advance to avoid them as much as possible (see the chart on page 29).

 At lunch one Friday, Ron and his friends began talking about having too little time to exercise. They decided that it would be fun to walk together. There was a nice park near the office, so the four friends decided to try to walk there together. The time that was convenient for most of them was during lunch on Monday, Wednesday, and Friday. Ron knew that getting away at lunchtime was sometimes difficult for him. But he decided to give it a try.

After lunch Friday, he went back to his office to check his schedule for the coming week. Unfortunately, his secretary had already scheduled lunch meetings with clients for all three of the days Ron and his friends had planned to walk. He really wanted to make time for walks, so he decided to make some adjustments to his schedule. He asked his secretary to reschedule his Friday appointment so he could walk with his friends that day. He penciled in time on Monday to take a short walk in the middle of the afternoon. He got up early Wednesday morning and walked before work.

Ron also looked at his calendar for the next month. He found at least two days each week during which he could block out time for walks with his friends during lunch. He also penciled in a walk before or after work on another day of the week.

You'll find that it's easy to avoid some lapses, hard to avoid others. Take, for example, the December holidays. It's easy to get caught up in the flurry of activities and commitments and let your physical activity habits fall by the wayside. But since you know these holidays come at the same time every year, you can plan ways to prevent these lapses and relapses. With an effective and realistic plan in place, you should be able to continue regular walking during the holidays. For example, instead of walking before work, you may want to walk at the mall for 20 to 30 minutes before starting your holiday shopping.

Use the table below to help you identify your particular high-risk situations and your plans for coping with them. Use some of the techniques and strategies we discussed, such as setting realistic goals, tracking your progress, recruiting help, thinking positively, and rewarding yourself.

Lapse Attack Plan

| High-Risk Situation | Can This Be . . . | | Plans |
	. . . Avoided?	. . . Coped With?	
Example: *Rain*	*No*	*Yes*	*Buy a poncho with a hood and an extra pair of walking shoes.*
Working late	*Sometimes*	*Yes*	*Walk in a.m. or get to work early*

In the beginning you'll get lots of urges to forego your walking. You'll tell yourself, "I don't feel like walking. I'll do it tomorrow." These urges can creep up without warning, so you need to be alert to them.

Typically, these urges start as a subtle awareness that you want to skip your walking. As you begin to pay attention to the urge, it grows stronger and stronger. Eventually, the urge may pass. The best thing to do is to have a plan in place to keep yourself from focusing on the urge. That will make it easier for you to outlast it.

The only time of day that Blanca can realistically walk is early in the morning before work. But she struggles with it almost every day. When the alarm goes off, she hits the snooze button. That's when the urge to skip her walk starts. As she lies there waiting for the alarm to go off again, the urge grows. Most of the time she gives in to it.

To combat the urge, Blanca got a new alarm clock without a snooze button. Now, the night before she plans to walk, she puts her walking clothes in the bathroom down the hall. This gets her out of her bedroom (so she's not tempted to crawl back into bed), and it keeps her up because she has to walk down the hall to get to her clothes. By the time she's dressed, she's wide awake and ready to head out the door.

WHEN YOU HAVE A LAPSE

Despite your best effort to prevent lapses, sometimes they do occur. When that happens to you, keep the following important things in mind.

- ☐ *Accept that a lapse is bound to happen sometime.* It does no good to beat yourself up for something you can't control or for making a mistake. If possible, remove yourself from the situation that triggered the lapse.
- ☐ *Coping is everything.* The way you cope with and manage a lapse is more important than the lapse itself. Don't berate yourself for having a lapse. Instead, set a small goal to achieve by the end of the day (for example, walk around the block). No matter how small, it will help you get back on track.
- ☐ *Make the most of it.* Think of the lapse as an opportunity to learn how you can minimize the risk of lapses in the future. Review the events that preceded the lapse and try to find out what occurred that could have triggered it. Then develop strategies to combat the triggers.

Are We Having Fun Yet?

Even with all the walking tools in the world, you probably won't stick with your walking plan unless it's fun. If walking is a chore, you'll drop it eventually. It's up to you to use your creativity to make walking a part of your life you really enjoy. Here are some helpful tactics you might consider.

- ☐ *Walk with other people.* Invite your family, friends, or neighbors along on your walk. They can keep you company and help you problem-solve along the way. Or join a walking club to make new friends and learn more about walking techniques.
- ☐ *Walk to music with a good beat.* Bring along a tiny sports radio and step to the beat of the music. Try marches, classics, even country and western. But if you're walking in a congested area, be sure you can still hear traffic sounds.
- ☐ *Listen to a book.* If you're an avid reader, you can now walk and read at the same time. Get a book on audiotape, pop it in a portable player, and go, go, go! Public libraries and some videotape rental stores have lots of books on tape.
- ☐ *Vary your walks.* If you walk in your neighborhood during the week, then find a different place to walk on weekends. Try different routes in your neighborhood or another neighborhood nearby. It's a great way to get landscaping ideas!
- ☐ *Play games on your walks.* For example, count how many different kinds of birds you see. Can you identify them by their song?
- ☐ *Take walking vacations.* Include walking as part of any trip or vacation you take. You'll see a lot more on foot than from a car or bus—and you can mingle with the natives!

These tips will help keep walking fresh and appealing. As you become more committed to being a physically active person, the tips and strategies described above will not be as necessary, because walking will have become a part of who you are. And no matter what happens, you'll have the confidence and drive to keep walking as a part of your life—for life.

CHAPTER

9

Advanced Walking

So you've completed several months of a basic walking program and you're now ready to add new skills to your routine. Several types of walking can increase the intensity of your workout and move you to a higher fitness level.

Some of these techniques require special equipment, such as hand weights, walking poles, or resistive cords. These devices can be fun and effective if you use them properly and don't let them slow your pace too much. If you prefer to walk unencumbered, you can try other advanced techniques, such as treadmill walking, stair-climbing, or race walking. You may even want to make the transition to jogging.

Hand Weights

Bored with regular walking? Then take it another step. Try power walking. That's brisk walking while holding hand weights. Power walking is perfect for people who want to increase their workout intensity without increasing their walking pace. Hand weights exercise your arms, shoulders, back, and chest muscles. They raise your heart rate and cause you to burn a great deal more calories during your walk. You can also use the hand weights to build muscle strength by adding a few exercises after your walk.

Follow the guidelines given here for using hand weights safely while walking.

If you have high blood pressure, heart disease, or you're pregnant, check with your doctor before adding weights to your walking routine.

USING HAND WEIGHTS SAFELY

☐ When adding weights to your walking program, always walk on a level surface or flat terrain.

☐ As your hands and forearms grip the weights, you may experience a slight elevation in blood pressure. Grip the weights gently so you don't restrict blood flow.

☐ It's not just the weight that makes power walking so effective. Your arm swing is also critical. Your movement should be controlled and smooth. Pump your arms vigorously, but do not overextend your natural range of motion.

☐ Don't use ankle weights while walking or jogging. They increase the impact and put added stress on your knees and ankle joints.

☐ If you have orthopedic pain or an injury, be cautious about using weights. Start with short walks and light weights, then build up slowly, to avoid injuries to the shoulder or elbow. The hand weights should never exceed three to five pounds each, depending upon your size and strength.

HOW TO USE HAND WEIGHTS

You might want to try the following techniques without weights first, using a brisk walking stride. Add weights as you advance.

Pump and Walk. Overemphasize regular arm swings by swinging one hand toward your head while extending your other arm behind you. Keep your elbows slightly bent. Alternate arm pumps. Practice this technique a few times without weights.

Alternating Arm Curls. Hold both arms horizontally at shoulder height. Bend one arm at the elbow and bring the forearm in toward your chest with your palm in. Repeat, alternating arms. Keep your upper arms extended from your side and your elbows in a stationary position.

Punch and Walk. Alternately punch your arms forward straight ahead of the body at shoulder height. Keep your elbow pointing straight back with your knuckles forward. Pull your elbow back behind you with each step.

Walking Poles

If you've ever been skiing, hiking, or mountaineering, you've no doubt used ski poles to help you stay balanced while covering uneven terrain. Using poles while walking is a relatively new practice. The fitness benefit of adding poles depends entirely on the effort you expend. When you vigorously plant the poles alongside you as you step and then push back on the pole with each stride, you can burn significantly more calories.

You'll find that the technique for applying resistance with poles is quite different from the resistance added when walking with hand weights. You work different muscles, primarily those in your upper back, your triceps, and your abdominal muscles. Another advantage of using poles is that they reduce the impact on your legs by letting your upper body bear some of the weight.

Poles also come equipped with comfortable hand grips and wrist straps that allow you to keep your hands relaxed, reducing the gripping action that can elevate blood pressure. However, they must be carried and stored, which may be a disadvantage when traveling.

Poles can actually help you walk faster, rather than slowing your pace as hand weights do. On the other hand, it takes concentration to master this technique and keep up the pace.

Resistive Cords

Resistive cords are elastic cords threaded through a padded belt that you wear around your waist. At each end of the resistive cord is a wrist-wrap, which you attach to your wrist. While walking, you build muscle strength by swinging your arms against the resistance of the cords. When you want to stop using the cords, you unfasten the wrist-wraps and let the cords hang at your waist.

These cords provide significant resistance to your shoulder muscles, triceps, back, and chest. Because the motion alters your natural arm swing more than other devices—you'll find that it's one arm stroke to every two-step cadence—you probably won't want to use cords during your entire workout. It may take a few walking sessions to get the hang of resistance cords. There are several levels of resistance, so begin with the lowest resistance and progress gradually. One advantage of resistive cords is that they are lightweight and easy to carry and store.

Race Walking

In race walking, vigorous arm movements and accentuated hip movements help increase your speed and lengthen your stride. Race walking is an advanced walking technique that requires special skill. It takes considerable concentration to synchronize the movement of the arms, trunk, and legs into a natural and harmonious gait. For that reason, you might benefit from coaching or lessons to help you master the technique.

Elite race walkers can move nearly as fast as some runners (six to seven miles per hour). Remember that there is some increased risk of injury due to the accentuated hip movement, so it's best to start with some supervision.

Walking/Jogging

If you're not interested in race walking but still want to pick up your pace without devices or equipment, consider a walk/jog routine. But before you do, be sure you don't have a condition that could be worsened by increasing impact and weight-bearing activity.

It's easy to combine walking and jogging. Here's how.

- □ *Vary the time.* Walk for 5 minutes, then jog for 5 minutes (or less). Repeat for a total of 30 minutes. Gradually increase the walking and jogging times to 10 minutes each and the total time to 40 minutes. You may want to stay with a walk/jog program or switch to all jogging. If jogging is your goal, gradually decrease the walking time and increase the jogging time.
- □ *Vary the distance.* Walk for ¼ mile, then jog for ¼ mile (or less). Repeat this pattern until you cover your distance goal.
- □ *Alternate the routine.* Walk one day and jog the next.

Treadmills and Stair-Climbing Machines

Treadmills allow you to exercise at a constant speed for a specified period of time. You can walk or jog on either a flat surface or an incline. You can increase intensity by increasing your walking speed or by elevating the deck of the treadmill.

Some treadmills are motorized; others are not. When walking on a non-motorized treadmill, you'll probably have to hold the handrail to maintain balance. This will limit your natural upper body walking or climbing movement and therefore decrease your aerobic benefit. Walking on a motorized treadmill allows more natural movements of your body and arms. If you hold the handrail, increase your walking intensity to compensate for the loss of effort you would have gained from swinging your arms.

Like treadmills, stair-climbing machines offer a precise workout intensity. You can find these machines in health clubs and fitness centers. Some people even purchase home exercise machines rather than spending money on membership fees. It's a good idea to be sure you enjoy this type of workout and are likely to stick with it before making a major investment.

If you're exercising indoors on a treadmill or stair-climbing machine, be aware that your body temperature may rise at a more rapid rate than when exercising outdoors and you will perspire more. Consider placing a fan nearby as a source of air for cooling, and remember to drink plenty of water.

Walking can be as simple and relaxing as a stroll in the park or it can be a vigorous workout. The great thing about it is that you decide what's best for you. Walking with hand weights, race walking, and walking on a treadmill are just a few ways you can reach a higher level of fitness through walking—if that's your goal. Just remember to take it one step at a time and keep it fun.

CHAPTER

10

Balancing Your Fitness Program

When most people think of fitness, they conjure up visions of people running marathons, swimming the English Channel, or bicycling in the Tour de France. All of these are aerobic endurance activities. But other parts of being fit are also important. As you age, muscular strength and flexibility become as important to fitness as aerobic endurance. So how do you get the benefits of all the components of fitness? By *varying* your physical activities. That gives you not just one kind of fitness, but *balanced* fitness.

Balanced fitness includes aerobic endurance, muscular strength and endurance, and flexibility. Aerobic endurance that comes from walking, running, swimming, and bicycling, for example, allows you to be active for an extended period without tiring. Flexibility, on the other hand, is when your muscles, limbs, and joints can move freely and completely without stiffness. Yoga and other stretching exercises can help with flexibility. Then there's muscular strength and endurance, which allow your muscles to maintain force. Weightlifting is one way to achieve this. Working out in each of these areas leads to balanced fitness.

If you watch a ballet dancer, you'll see a good example of balanced fitness at work. Ballet dancers must have the aerobic endurance to practice long hours and perform night after night. They must also have great strength to dance *en pointe* and to perform leaps and other difficult moves. And they must be super flexible to deliver a smooth, supple performance.

By contrast, bodybuilders concentrate mainly on strength-building activities to develop great muscle mass. But if they neglect aerobic exercise and flexibility training altogether, they wind up with strong but rigid muscles. Fortunately, many training programs for bodybuilders now include flexibility exercises, which make it easier to develop and execute posing routines. Many programs also include aerobic training, which can improve muscular definition while reducing body fat.

To achieve balanced fitness, you need to exercise in a way that addresses each of the three concerns. If you're just starting a walking program, go ahead and concentrate on building your aerobic endurance. Give yourself a chance to first make walking a way of life. Then slowly add other aerobic, strength-training, and flexibility activities, especially when you feel yourself becoming "stale" or bored with walking. (You may need to get more information before beginning any strength-training or flexibility activities. A good place to start is your community center, local Y, or fitness center.)

The Joys of Heavy Breathing

Aerobic activities challenge your heart and lungs by using the large muscle groups in a rhythmic manner for an extended period of time. And walking certainly fits the bill. In fact, plenty of activities qualify as aerobic. Swimming, bicycling, running, roller-blading, cross-country skiing, and stair-climbing are all aerobic activities. Also, vigorous lifestyle activities such as vacuuming, digging in the garden, and washing the car can be considered aerobic as well.

As you become more physically fit by walking, consider adding other aerobic activities to your routine. For example, instead of walking five days a week, you could try walking three days and bicycling two days. Adding other aerobic activities to your bag of exercise tricks is a good opportunity to resume old hobbies or develop new skills and interests.

Leaving Wimp City

Muscular strength is an important part of your overall well-being, even though it's not directly related to heart health. Each of us gradually loses muscular strength as we age. With this loss of strength we may tire more easily, become prone to injury, and, ultimately, become less able to function on our own.

Fortunately, you can dramatically slow down this loss of strength. Recent studies have shown that even elderly people can regain some of their muscular strength. How? By doing physical activities that challenge your muscles—by pushing them against some type of resistance, for example. One study showed strength improvements in elderly men and women (in their nineties!) after they completed an eight-week weight training program. Some improved enough to get out of a chair unassisted or walk without the aid of a cane.

Strength-building activities can also help you reduce the risk of injury, prevent osteoporosis, and improve posture. So what *are* strength-building activities? Weightlifting is one. Another is calisthenics, such as push-ups, pull-ups, and sit-ups. Others include certain types of martial arts, lifting or carrying heavy objects, and exercising in water. As with walking, start slowly. If you haven't been training, get information from a reputable source, and remember to start with very light weights to build endurance.

Strength-Building Activities

Weightlifting
- Free Weights
  - ☐ Barbells
  - ☐ Dumbbells
  - ☐ Light weights from around the house (books, filled cans, etc.)
- Resistance Machines

Calisthenics
- Heel Raises
- Lunges
- Pull-ups
- Push-ups
- Sit-ups

Other
- Backpacking with a heavy pack*
- Digging*
- Martial Arts
- Rock Climbing*
- Snow Shoveling*
- Water Aerobics*

*May also improve aerobic fitness if done continuously for five minutes or longer.

Samson's Secret

Building strength is not just for football players and bodybuilders. Including muscular strength and endurance activities in a balanced fitness program can improve your walking performance, too.

THE BENEFITS OF STRENGTH-BUILDING

☐ *Boosts upper-body strength.* For the most part, you don't use the muscles in your upper body (neck and chest) during walking. However, weak muscles in these areas can hinder your walking enjoyment and performance. Have your shoulders and neck ever been sore after a long walk? Or would you like to increase your walking pace? If you improve the strength and endurance of your upper-body muscles, they'll be better able to withstand the stress of a long walk. These improvements will also allow you to use your arms more vigorously, so that you can pick up your pace.

☐ *Prevents common overuse injuries.* While walking is safe, your knees, lower back, and feet can still get sore. You can reduce this risk of injury if you strengthen the muscles that support and surround these areas.

☐ *Improves muscle symmetry.* When you do only one type of aerobic activity, some muscles will develop while others will weaken. Over time, this imbalance can lead to injury. If you add strength training, you can build the weaker muscles for a more effective and efficient overall result.

☐ *Improves your fitness level.* Strength training can challenge your muscles and bones in ways that walking can't. It can boost your overall fitness level beyond what you can accomplish by just walking. It can also help your walking performance—you will walk faster and longer.

STRENGTH TRAINING RULES

How do you build strength? From weightlifting machines to rubber bands to calisthenics, there are many ways to challenge your muscles. But each method uses the following basic principles.

☐ **Overload.** You need to challenge your muscles with overload. They'll eventually get stronger in an effort to adapt to that overload or stress. Conversely, if you don't challenge your muscles, they'll gradually grow weaker and atrophy.

☐ **Progression.** As with aerobic activity, you need to start at a comfortable level and gradually add additional stress to your muscles. As you get stronger, the activity will become easier. To continue building strength, you will need to gradually add more resistance or weight.

☐ *Specificity.* You must work the specific muscles you want to improve. Obviously, you can't build strength in your arms if you do only lower body exercise.

Jock Talk

■ "Rep" is short for *repetition.* In weight training it refers to the number of times a muscle contracts without resting. If you lift a barbell 10 times in a row, you've done 10 reps.

■ "Set" refers to a group of repetitions performed in sequence; there is a brief period of rest between sets for muscles to recover.

Regardless of the strength-building method you use, a beginning program usually has these features:

☐ Works 8 to 12 different large muscle groups
☐ Includes 8 to 12 reps per set. If you can't do at least 8 reps, reduce the weight or resistance. If you can do more than 12 reps comfortably, increase the weight or resistance slightly.
☐ Uses one to three sets per muscle group

Warm-ups and cool-downs are important in a strength-building program. A warm-up for weightlifting purposes may simply consist of one set of each exercise (8 to 10 reps) using 50 to 60 percent of the weight load you will use in your training session. Strength-building activities won't directly help your heart, but they are an important part of maintaining a healthy body and general well-being, especially as you get older.

Limber Up for Life

If there's stress in your life, you may have low-back pain, stiff neck muscles, and tight shoulder muscles. Or maybe your job—whether it involves lifting or sitting at a desk—leaves you with sore shoulders and a stiff neck. In fact, many people have chronically tight muscles, ligaments, and tendons. These symptoms can drastically reduce their body movements and sometimes cause chronic pain. For example, tightness in your lower back muscles, buttocks, and the back of your thighs (called hamstring muscles) can create low-back pain.

Physical activities that promote flexibility by helping you move the different parts of your body freely, through their full range of motion, are important. They help counteract the natural tendency to lose your flexibility and suppleness as you age. Flexibility exercises can be important steps along the way to top-notch health.

A light aerobic warm-up to increase your circulation is ideal before doing yoga or stretching exercises. For example, you may want to walk at a moderate pace for 3 to 5 minutes followed by 15 to 25 jumping jacks to increase your heart rate.

Oh, My Aching Back!

Low-back pain is the number one cause of absenteeism and workman's compensation claims.

WARM-UPS ARE HOT

Stretching can help your body become more flexible. Like strength-building activities, stretching doesn't reduce your risk of heart disease. But when you reduce your muscle tension and increase the range of motion in your joints and muscles, you can help limit soreness and stiffness. That way, you can get the most out of your heart-protecting aerobic activities. Stretching is also a good way to cool down after vigorous activity.

For example, it is a good idea to stretch your back and leg muscles after you walk. You can also stretch while sitting at work. Neck stiffness is a common complaint at the worksite, and "stretching breaks" can help alleviate this stiffness. Finally, maintaining loose and limber muscles and joints can help you maintain good posture. You'll find stretching techniques and activities to enhance your walking program on pages 66–71. You may want to try renting a yoga or stretching video or taking a class at your local community center or Y.

One last hint: If possible, periodically treat yourself to a massage. Massaging muscles stimulates the blood flow to the muscle area. This increased blood flow can help heal muscle fibers that get damaged as a natural part of increased physical activity. Of course, muscle massage by itself won't improve your flexibility, but it may boost the results of your regular stretching program. Besides, it's a great way to relax.

Putting Balanced Fitness Into Your Future

Now it's time to plan a balanced fitness program for yourself. Use the Balanced Fitness Assessment below to jump-start your thinking. You'll begin with walking, of course, then add other activities to round out your plan. Write your responses in the space provided.

Balanced Fitness Assessment

1. What physical activities or sports have you enjoyed doing in the past?
➤ _____
➤ _____
➤ _____

2. What new activities would you like to try?
➤ _____
➤ _____
➤ _____

3. What activities, facilities, or equipment are currently available to you—
   At home?
➤ _____
➤ _____

   At work?
➤ _____
➤ _____

   In the neighborhood or local community?
➤ _____
➤ _____

In the table below, organize all the activities you listed above in their proper column. Then circle one or two activities in each column.

Covering the Fitness Bases

Aerobic Endurance Activities	Strength-Building Activities	Flexibility Activities
Example: *Walking*	*Hand weights*	*Yoga*

Complete the chart below using the aerobic endurance, strength-building, and flexibility activities you circled above.

My Total Fitness Plan

Days of Week	Fitness Component*	Physical Activity
Monday, Wednesday, and Friday	■ Aerobic endurance ■ Strength-building	■ ■
Tuesday	■ Aerobic endurance ■ Special flexibility activity	■ ■
Thursday	Rest	
Weekends	■ Aerobic endurance ■ Depends on activity	■ ■ Recreational, lifestyle or sport activities.

*Basic stretching activities should be included in the warm-up and cool-down phases of any aerobic endurance or strength-building activity.

Use this assessment to help you start planning a balanced fitness program. If the activity you selected is new to you, spend some time learning the skills and techniques associated with it. You may be able to find information at your local library or community center. Or contact a personal trainer for a few instructional sessions.

CHAPTER

11

Eating for Health and Fitness

You don't have to be a rocket scientist to know how to eat right.

Unfortunately, some people think you do. The media constantly reports conflicting nutrition studies that can confuse consumers until they give up trying to understand good nutrition.

But here's some good news: Nutrition isn't about what you can't or shouldn't eat. Rather, it's a simple message of knowing what to eat, how much to eat, and planning ahead so that over time your food habits are pretty consistent, at least 80 percent of the time.

Taking Good Nutrition in Stride

Volumes have been written on nutrition. But the simple pyramid, on the next page, includes just about everything you need to know to choose a healthful diet. All your favorite foods fit somewhere into this Healthy Heart Food Pyramid. The problem is that many Americans read the pyramid upside down.

As you can see, the foundation for heart-healthy eating is a diet that includes lots of breads, cereals, pasta, and starchy vegetables—with plenty of fruits and vegetables. Low-fat dairy products, then lean meat, poultry, and fish, are next in priority. Last and least are fats, oils, nuts, and sweets. You'll want to go easy on those. To get the nutrients you need, it's important to select a wide variety of foods. At the same time, you need the appropriate number of calories to maintain a healthy weight. So while your favorite food may fit in the pyramid, look closely: You may have to cut back on your serving size.

The Healthy Heart Food Pyramid

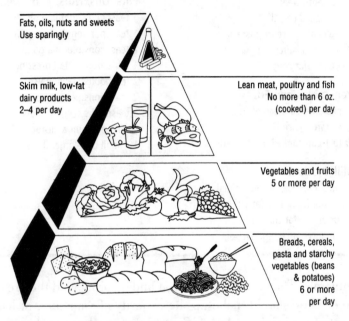

Fats, oils, nuts and sweets
Use sparingly

Skim milk, low-fat
dairy products
2–4 per day

Lean meat, poultry and fish
No more than 6 oz.
(cooked) per day

Vegetables and fruits
5 or more per day

Breads, cereals,
pasta and starchy
vegetables (beans
& potatoes)
6 or more
per day

- The American Heart Association has adapted the Food Guide Pyramid, developed by the U.S. Dept. of Agriculture and U.S. Dept. of Health and Human Services, to be consistent with the AHA Dietary Guidelines for Healthy American Adults.
- Limit your sodium intake to no more than 3,000 milligrams per day.
- Eat no more than 3–4 egg yolks per week. (Egg whites are not limited.)

BUILDING A GOOD FOUNDATION WITH CARBOHYDRATES

Carbohydrates provide calories that fuel your muscles and brain. Carbohydrate-rich foods include breads, grains, fruits, and vegetables.

There are two kinds of carbohydrates: *complex* carbohydrates and *simple* carbohydrates. Complex carbohydrates are grain products, like bread, cereal, pasta, potatoes, and rice as well as vegetables. Simple carbohydrates are basically sweet foods, including sugar, honey, desserts, and soft drinks. Fruit contains both types of carbohydrates.

Typically, complex carbohydrates are rich in fiber, vitamins, and

---

What Is One Serving?

Breads, Cereals, Pasta, and Starchy Vegetables
1 slice bread
¼ cup nugget or bud-type cereal
½ cup hot cereal
1 cup flaked cereal
1 cup cooked rice or pasta
¼ to ½ cup starchy vegetables
1 cup low-fat soup

Vegetables and Fruits
1 medium-size piece of fruit
½ cup fruit juice
½ to 1 cup cooked or raw vegetables

Milk Products
1 cup skim, ½%, or 1% fat milk
1 cup nonfat or low-fat yogurt
1 ounce low-fat cheese
½ cup low-fat cottage cheese

Meat, Poultry, and Fish
3 ounces cooked (4 ounces raw) lean meat,
    poultry, or fish

Fats, Oils, Nuts, and Sweets
1 teaspoon vegetable oil
1 teaspoon regular margarine
2 teaspoons diet margarine
1 tablespoon salad dressing
2 teaspoons mayonnaise
2 teaspoons peanut butter
3 teaspoons seeds or nuts
⅛ of a medium avocado
10 small or 5 large olives

---

minerals. They are also low in fat and calories, and they're cholesterol free. They should make up the majority of your diet, at least 50 percent of your daily calories. Simple carbohydrate foods such as cakes, cookies, and pastries tend to be low in nutrients and high in calories. Many people, including athletes, think these foods are rich in carbohydrates. What they don't realize is that 60 to 70 percent of the calories in these foods often come from fat. Such foods should make up only about 10 percent of your daily calories.

FAT FACTS—THE GOOD, THE BAD, AND THE UGLY

Fat provides energy for the body. It also adds flavor to our food and makes us feel satisfied after eating. That's good.

The problem with fat is that many people eat far too much of it. The American Heart Association recommends that less than 30 percent of your daily calories come from fat. Yet, for the average American, fat intake is about 34 percent of those calories. A major concern is that high intakes of fat, especially saturated fat, are strongly linked to heart disease.

When you look closely at fat, you'll find that all fats are *not* created equal. Oh, they all contain lots of calories, but they do not have the same effect on your body.

Fats can be divided into two main types—saturated and unsaturated. Saturated fat is found mostly in foods of animal origin and in certain plant oils (palm, coconut, hydrogenated vegetable). Saturated fat causes blood cholesterol levels to climb. Unsaturated fats include polyunsaturated and monounsaturated fats. Polyunsaturated fats are found in vegetable oils like corn oil, safflower oil, sunflower oil, soybean oil, etc. Monounsaturated fats are found in canola oil, olive oil, and peanut oil. Unsaturated fats help to lower blood cholesterol levels when they are substituted for saturated fat. Monounsaturated fats can actually help lower LDL cholesterol levels. LDL cholesterol is often called the "bad cholestrol" because it is strongly associated with an increased risk of heart disease.

Of course, everyone needs *some* fat. The best thing is to aim for a low-fat—not a NO-fat—diet. You need some fat to help your body absorb fat-soluble vitamins and to help your body produce hormones, but you should be careful not to overdo it.

NO BONES ABOUT IT—LOW-FAT DAIRY PRODUCTS ARE TERRIFIC

Everyone needs calcium. Children and teens need it for growth, and adults need it to maintain strong bones. But you don't need the fat that comes with whole-milk dairy products. Fortunately, you can get your calcium without the fat. Just trade in your whole-milk dairy products for low-fat ones. Then make it a point to include them in your diet as long as you live.

If low-fat is good, isn't skim milk even better? The following table will show you the huge difference in today's dairy offerings.

Milk-Fat Made Easy

Type of Milk	Grams of Fat in 1 Cup	% Fat by Weight	% Fat by Calories
Whole milk	8 grams	3.5	48
2% Low-fat milk	5 grams	2	38
1% Low-fat milk	2 grams	1	28
Skim milk	trace	trace	4

Remember, the American Heart Association recommends that your total fat intake be less than 30 percent of your total daily calories. So skim milk and 1% fat milk fit perfectly into a healthy diet.

The only difference between a glass of whole milk and a glass of skim milk is the fat, but it is a *big* difference. The 8 grams of fat in a cup of whole milk is equivalent to two pats of butter, and most of the fat is saturated fat. Skim milk, by comparison, has virtually no fat yet all the calcium of whole milk. So by switching to skim and 1% low-fat milk, you are cutting back on one of the major sources of saturated fat in the diet.

PROTEIN POWER: LEAN MEAT, POULTRY, AND FISH

When it comes to protein, think "lean." Lean cuts of beef and pork, skinless poultry, and all fish and seafood fit into a healthy eating plan. And serving sizes should be modest. In fact, the ideal serving size of meat is 3 ounces cooked, or about the size of a deck of cards. For top physical fitness and heart health, the American Heart Association recommends no more than two servings for a maximum total of 6 ounces cooked meat a day.

Many Americans are learning to use meat as a light touch in planning diets that are low in fat. Consider meat a condiment or a side dish. Meat, chicken, and fish complement many pasta and rice dishes. Just compare your dinner plate to the Healthy Heart Food Pyramid (page 111). Two-thirds of your plate should be covered with starches, vegetables, and fruits. Add a glass of low-fat or skim milk on the side. Bon appetit!

How to Walk All Over Fat

If you're like most people, you'd like to lose a little weight. The truth is, America's national waistline is expanding. More people than ever before are fighting the battle of the bulge. In fact, one in three adults are overweight (that is, they're 20 percent or more above their ideal weight). If you find yourself in this category, take heart. You're not alone. And here's good news: Walking could be the key to your success for long-term weight loss.

THE CALORIE BALANCING ACT

Weight control is not easy. Genetic factors and behavior patterns complicate the issue. Still, the amount of calories you consume mainly determines your body weight and body composition.

If the calories you eat equal the number of calories you use for basic living and physical activity, you'll maintain your present weight. You'll lose weight when you expend more calories than you take in. No adult should eat less than 1,200 calories a day. Diets of less than 1,200 calories simply don't provide enough nutrients; they should only be practiced under strict medical supervision. So the secret of permanent weight loss is eating a nutritious, low-calorie diet and getting plenty of regular exercise.

WEIGHT LOSS WITHOUT EXERCISE? FAT CHANCE!

You've heard it before, and we'll say it again, "Diets don't work." In fact, experts estimate that 95 percent of any weight loss is regained—unless regular exercise is included in a maintainance program. Severe dieting often leads to binge eating. Fasting or extreme calorie restriction causes the body to lose water and lean muscle. What actually happens when people lose ten to fifteen pounds or more in a one- to two-week period? Some experts estimate that more than 70 percent of the weight loss is water loss and more than 20 percent is lean body tissue. That leaves only 3 percent to 5 percent of the weight loss as fat. No wonder people using these regimens feel so bad! Also, the loss of muscle that occurs causes your metabolism to slow down, which is *not* what you need.

Your extra body fat didn't accumulate overnight. So it won't disappear overnight, either. Experts say that you should aim to lose no more than one-half to two pounds per week by eating less and exercising more (See page 13 for calorie expenditures for a 30-Minute Workout.) When you walk every day, you burn a lot of calories in a week.

So how much exercise do you need to lose weight? Well, that depends how often you exercise and for how long at a time. To lose the most weight and keep injuries to bones, joints, and muscles low, you'll need to do low-intensity exercises more often and for longer stretches. While exercising three times a week is great for cardiovascular fitness, you may have to exercise nearly every day to lose weight.

In 15 minutes of brisk walking, you use enough energy to burn the calories in. . . .

- ☐ 10 potato chips
- ☐ ⅓ cup ice cream
- ☐ 2 cups of cantalope pieces
- ☐ 25 baby carrots (or three regular-size carrots)
- ☐ 1 cup (8 ounces) orange juice
- ☐ ½ cup frozen yogurt
- ☐ ½ medium baked potato
- ☐ ½ glazed doughnut
- ☐ ⅕ of a fast food specialty burger

As a rough guide, walkers can figure expending 100 calories per mile. It will be slightly less for thin people or slower-paced walkers; slightly more for heavier people or faster-paced walkers.

HAVE YOUR CAKE—AND EAT IT, TOO

Staying fit, trim, and healthy is easier than you think. Just remember that all foods fit somewhere into a healthy eating plan. Use the food pyramind to help you choose the kinds of foods you want to eat every day. Fill up on complex carbohydrates like grains, legumes, fruits, and vegetables. Add low-fat and nonfat dairy products. Make protein a modest part of your meal—not the main event. Finally, go easy on fats and oils. When you balance your calorie intake and energy output, you'll find that eating this way helps your waistline as well as your heart.

12

Injuries Are a Pain

One of the great advantages of walking is that it is usually safe. Still, injuries can occur. The most common cause of injury for walkers is doing too much too soon or working too hard for too long.

An Ounce of Prevention, a Pound of Cure: R-I-C-E

To prevent walking injuries:

☐ Start slowly and increase gradually.
☐ Wear properly fitted shoes.
☐ Perform stretching and strength-building exercises regularly.

If you *do* get an injury, apply the R-I-C-E principle: Rest, Ice, Compression, and Elevation.

REST   Reduce or discontinue activity as soon as you no-
                tice the injury. If you continue to walk, you may
                aggravate the injury.
ICE   Ice is the most effective, safest, and cheapest form
                of treating an exercise injury. Apply an ice pack
                immediately. Ice decreases swelling and blood
                flow and reduces pain. If there is swelling, con-

tinue to apply the ice pack intermittently for 72 hours. *Don't* apply ice directly to the skin, where it can be irritating; first wrap the ice or ice pack in a cloth. Apply it for no more than 20 minutes. Then allow the tissue to return to normal temperature for several minutes and apply ice again for up to 20 minutes. *Don't* apply the ice for longer than 20 minutes at a time.

COMPRESSION   Wrap the injury in an elastic bandage firmly but not tight enough to cut off the circulation. During the early stages when swelling is severe, loosen the wrap every half hour, then reapply it. Compression reduces swelling.

ELEVATION   At first, elevate the injured limb so that it's higher than the heart at all times (including during sleep), until swelling has subsided. In this way, gravity prevents the pooling of blood and other fluids.

If the pain is severe, if you cannot move the injured part, or if the injury does not seem to be healing after reasonable home treatment, see a physician immediately.

Sweet Relief!

Over-the-counter pain relievers and anti-inflammatories such as aspirin or ibuprofin can help ease the pain and reduce inflammation of minor sprains and strains. Acetaminophen is better for relief of muscle soreness.

The table on pages 120–121 gives information about some specific injuries a walker might encounter.

Illness and Exercise Don't Mix

Everyone catches a cold at one time or another. The symptoms vary but usually include one or more of the following: coughing, sneezing, a runny nose, a sore and scratchy throat, aching muscles, a low-grade fever, and/or malaise (the blahs). You may not sleep well.

You may not have much of an appetite. At a time like this, should you exercise?

The symptoms of a cold are a sign that your body is fighting a virus. Bed rest will not cure a cold or even relieve the symptoms. If you feel up to it, there's no harm in exercising. Just cut back on the intensity and duration of your usual walk. Never force yourself to exercise if you feel too tired or unfit. And don't exercise if you have a fever.

Taking Care of Yourself

1. Engage in only limited, mild exercise when suffering from a minor illness such as a cold or the flu.
2. Do not exercise if you have a fever. Do not resume exercise until you have been free of fever for at least 24 hours.
3. After an illness, exercise at a lower intensity for shorter periods to avoid over-taxing the body and to give your body a chance to adapt as you resume your previous activities.

You will occasionally get sick. Disruptions to your exercise plans will occur. Expect them and plan how you will overcome these circumstances. A break of two or three days in your exercise program isn't much of a setback. Even if an illness lingers, don't despair, and by all means, don't throw in the towel.

It's important to realize that trying to exercise during recovery from an injury or illness can set you back further than not exercising. Be patient when trying to make your comeback. After you are feeling better, start slowly by walking less than your usual time for a few days or a couple of weeks until you're feeling back up to snuff.

Injury Treatment Tactics

Injury Location	If you feel . . .	It could be . . .	Recommended Treatment	Prevention
Foot	Pain in the bottom of the foot through the arch and heel; pain in the morning but feels better when you walk on it	Plantar Fasciitis	• R-I-C-E • Non-weight-bearing activities such as swimming, cycling • Arch support • Shortened stride • Orthotics • Anti-inflammatory medication	• Stretch calf and Achilles tendon. • Use adequate arch support in shoes. • Limit high-intensity activity on hard surfaces.
	Pain in the heel; may be swollen and bruised	Heel Bruise or Stone Bruise	• R-I-C-E • New shoes • Heel pad or cup • Don't walk barefoot • Anti-inflammatory medication	• Wear shoes with proper padding. • Walk on soft surfaces (grass instead of concrete).
	Pain in the heel that diminishes after walking for a few minutes	Heel Spur	• R-I-C-E • Heel pad or lift • Orthotics • Anti-inflammatory medication	• Wear shoes with proper arch support. • Reduce prolonged periods of standing.
	Pain in the ball of the foot right below the base of the big toe	Sesamoiditis	• R-I-C-E • See your doctor	• Reduce weight-bearing activities as soon as you feel pain.
	Pain on the surface of the toes	Corns	• Relieve pressure on the spot using special pads • New shoes if yours are too tight • Orthotics	• Make sure shoes fit correctly.
	Sharp pain that starts at the ball of the foot and shoots to the end of the toes	Morton's Neuroma	• R-I-C-E • Padding under the ball of the foot • See your doctor. (Surgery may be recommended.) • Anti-inflammatory medication	• Apply minimal impact on ball of foot. • Exercise only on soft surfaces. • Wear shoes of proper width.
	Pain on localized places on the skin	Blisters	• Wash area surrounding blister. Pierce edge of blister with sterilized needle. Leave skin in place. Place protective padding around blister. Be on the alert for signs of infection.	• Wear properly fitting socks and shoes.

Injury Location	If you feel . . .	It could be . . .	Recommended Treatment	Prevention
Shin	Pain in the front of side of the lower leg	Many different possible causes	• R-I-C-E • Orthotics • Calf stretches and toe raises • Anti-inflammatory medication	• Wear shoes with proper shock absorption. • Do calf stretches and toe raises.
Calf	Tenderness and pain in the lower calf and back of the ankle	Achilles Tendonitis	• R-I-C-E • Stretching of calf muscles • Anti-inflammatory medication	• Do stretching exercises. • Wear shoes that help keep your foot from rotating inward as you walk.
Knee	Pain and stiffness when walking stairs; grating sensation as knee joint is bent; general pain in kneecap area	Chondromalacia	• R-I-C-E • Reduce walking distance • Walk on soft surface • Strengthen muscles in front of thigh and stretch muscles in back of thigh • Anti-inflammatory medication	• Wear shoes with good arch support.
	Pain inside the knee; swelling in front and behind the knee; difficulty moving the knee joint	Cartilage tears	• R-I-C-E • See your doctor. (Surgery may be needed.)	• Maintain strength in the muscle around the knee joint. • Limit sharp, twisting motions. • Use care when walking on uneven surfaces.
Other Joints	Pain and stiffness with movement	Bursitis or Tendonitis	• R-I-C-E • Anti-inflammatory medication	• Gradually adapt to increased activity levels.
	Severe pain and swelling, usually in ankles and knees	Damage to ligaments (i.e., sprain) usually caused by twisting and sharp turning	• R-I-C-E • Depending on severity, medical attention may be needed. See your doctor.	• Build up the muscle around the joint to better support extreme forces.

Special Cases

If you're eager to begin a walking program but you have a challenging medical condition such as heart disease, arthritis, or diabetes, or if you're pregnant or obese, don't worry. People with these conditions manage to walk every day, and so can you.

We've prepared some helpful walking and exercise hints that cover the needs and problems of several specific medical conditions. Experience has shown that when you simply take a few precautions, you can easily participate in a regular walking program.

As always, though, check with your doctor before beginning any exercise program.

Walking for a Problem-Free Pregnancy

Moderate exercise is great for most pregnant women. If you're already active, you can continue your regular exercise program during pregnancy if your doctor gives the okay. As a general rule, it's best to stick with your usual exercise program or moderate it with appropriate alternatives during pregnancy. For example, many women runners combine walking and running in the beginning of the pregnancy and then make a transition to a walking program four or five months into the pregnancy.

If you're not active but want to begin an exercise program while you're pregnant, low-intensity walking is a great way to start. Increase your activity level very slowly and check out other alternatives, like water walking (see pages 130–132).

Walking During Pregnancy Can . . .

☐ Reduce tension and help you cope with the physical and emotional stresses of pregnancy
☐ Improve your sleep despite the discomfort of an enlarged stomach
☐ Help reduce constipation, which can be a real problem for pregnant women
☐ Speed up your recovery after childbirth
☐ Improve postpartum muscle tone

WALKING GUIDELINES WHEN YOU'RE PREGNANT

☐ Your exercise sessions should be regular. Try to walk at a low or moderate pace at least three or four times a week for a *total* of 30 minutes per day. Limit strenuous activity to 15 minutes at a time.

☐ Drink plenty of water before and after walking. Remember that you need to drink more water than usual to meet the fluid needs of your baby. Drinking water during any form of physical activity helps avoid the dehydration and elevated body temperature that could injure a developing baby.

☐ Your body temperature should never exceed 100 degrees F (38 degrees C). If it's a hot day, take it *slow*.

☐ Don't exceed a heart rate of 140 beats per minute. (See page 42 for an explanation of how to check your heart rate.) Be sure you recover to your pre-walk heart rate within fifteen minutes of your walking session.

☐ Warming up and cooling down are important (see pages 66–71). During pregnancy your muscles and joints are looser than usual, so stretch carefully.

☐ After your fourth month of pregnancy, don't exercise at all while lying on your back, such as in sit-ups. This can block the blood supply to your uterus and lower the fetal heart rate.

☐ If you need to rest during or just after your walk, lie down on your side, not on your back.

Walking for Heart Patients

The American Heart Association estimates that about 11.7 million Americans have coronary heart disease. Each year about 1.5 million people have heart attacks, and almost one-third are fatal.

Staying physically active plays a key role in preventing heart disease. It is also one of the key components in any cardiac rehabilitation program. Exercise helps heart patients recover after a heart attack, bypass surgery, or balloon angioplasty. Ideally, a heart patient should start with a hospital-based cardiac rehabilitation program within a few weeks of being discharged from the hospital. A good rehabilitation program offers exercise training, nutrition education, psychological counseling, vocational counseling, and risk factor modification.

Controllable Risk Factors for Heart Attack and Stroke

☐ Cigarette and tobacco smoke
☐ High cholesterol (200 milligrams per deciliter or greater)
☐ High blood pressure
☐ Physical inactivity

Contributing Factors for Heart Attack and Stroke

☐ Diabetes
☐ Obesity
☐ Individual response to stress

How Exercise Helps Your Heart

☐ Helps restore optimum work, daily living, and lifestyle status
☐ Improves fitness and builds muscular strength and endurance
☐ Reduces cardiovascular risk factors, including high cholesterol and high blood pressure

WALKING FOR REHAB: WHAT TO KNOW BEFORE YOU GO

☐ Before starting your walking program, be sure to get your doctor's okay. People with heart disease are not all alike: You may need supervision during exercise training, or you may be able to walk, and even jog, independently.

☐ If you have coronary artery disease, it's important to determine your target heart rate. Because certain cardiac medications (such as beta blockers) lower the heart rate both at rest and during exercise, the target rate test on pages 42–44 may not be accurate. Instead, your doctor may perform certain tests to determine your target heart rate.

☐ Consider wearing a heart rate monitor. It will help you stay within your target heart rate, which is the safe and beneficial intensity range for cardiovascular health. If you're below your target heart rate, walk faster. If you're above your target heart rate, *slow down.*

☐ Always cool down after exercise by walking very slowly, allowing the heart rate to return to its resting rate.

☐ Avoid walking in extremely cold and extremely hot environments.

☐ Drink water before, during, and after walking.

☐ Stop walking if you feel pain or discomfort in your chest, abdomen, neck, or jaw; tightness in your chest; pain radiating down your left arm; shortness of breath; or nausea. These could be warning signs that the heart is not getting enough oxygen. Contact your doctor immediately.

 When Jim was 45 years old, he had a heart attack. He told his doctor that it felt like an elephant was sitting on his chest. While he was recuperating in the hospital, Jim thought about his lifestyle over the past several years. Although he had played basketball in college, he had completely dropped all physical activity since. His only form of exercise was walking to the coffee room at the office several times a day. He knew he really didn't watch what he ate and he was a little overweight. When he thought about all of this, he realized how much he had neglected his health. The heart attack had been a serious shock.

When Jim was released from the hospital a short time later, his doctor referred him to a cardiac rehabilitation program. Three times a week for six weeks, Jim went to exercise class. He learned how to use light free-weights and to exercise on a treadmill, stationary bike, and rowing machine. Jim's wife Allison was delighted that he was attending rehabilitation classes where he would receive training and supervision.

During his six-week rehabilitation, Jim benefited from the social support of his fellow classmates and the education he received from his therapists. He left the program with a plan to walk four to five times a week. Now, instead of watching television in the evenings, Jim and Allison enjoy a three-mile walk around their neighborhood. Together, with the help of a dietician, they have restructured their diet and both have lost weight. Jim considers himself fortunate to have had a second chance to take care of his body and reduce the chances of a second heart attack.

_____

You're As Young As You Feel: Tips For Older Walkers

Your chronological age doesn't really mean much. What does matter is how old you feel. Many people who have been physically active throughout their lives feel younger than they are.

Too many people give up on physical activity as they grow older. Of course, that's the worst thing you can do. If you're inactive, you'll lose muscle fiber at a rate of 3 to 5 percent every decade after age 30. That's a 30 percent muscle fiber loss by age 60! At that rate, you'll eventually lose the ability to carry on the normal activities of daily living. The truth is, you must remain physically active to combat this loss of muscle and keep your independence. It's the "use it or lose it" principle in action.

Whatever your age, you can benefit from a walking program. If you're starting a walking program for the first time as an older person, check out the following suggestions. (For purposes of this discussion, an older person is a man over age 40 or a woman over age 50.)

OLDER WALKERS' CHECKLIST

☐ If you're older or if you have a family history of heart disease, check with your doctor first. It's a good idea to have a physical examination and take a graded exercise test before you start a strenuous walking program.

☐ Because muscular adaptation and elasticity is generally slowed with age, take a bit more time warming up and cooling down. Make sure you stretch slowly.

☐ Start exercising at a low intensity, especially if you have been mostly sedentary, and progress gradually.

☐ Make sure you drink water on a fixed schedule, especially when walking in hot, humid conditions. As you age, your sense of thirst tends to decrease and you can't completely rely on your own internal sense of thirst.

Obesity

If you're more than 20 percent overweight, you're considered obese. Many obese people do not follow a regular exercise program. If you're obese, one of your first goals should be to establish such a program, and walking's a great way to start. If you walk every day, you'll burn a lot of calories in a week. If you combine daily walking with a reduced-calorie diet, you have the best approach to weight loss.

If you're obese, you're at an increased risk of exercise-related injuries, because the extra weight puts more strain on your joints. Low-impact exercises such as walking are best. Just be sure to start your walking program gradually and progress slowly. At first, emphasize the duration and frequency of your exercise rather than its intensity. Walking in water that's waist or chest deep (see pages 130–132) can help you burn lots of calories with little risk of injury because it's nearly non-weight-bearing.

Walking for Obesity

☐ Aids fat loss
☐ Reduces blood pressure
☐ Lowers cholesterol and triglyceride levels
☐ Increases HDL levels
☐ Improves glucose tolerance
☐ Improves self-esteem

No matter what your condition or need, you can alter your walking techniques to make fitness possible. Your age and medical condition don't really matter. If you can walk at all, you can create a regular walking plan that will work for you.

How to Track Down Walking Opportunities

You walk around the local high school track every day. You walk the malls on Saturdays. And you take the stairs at work. That's good, but are you *really* taking advantage of every opportunity to add more walking to your day? This chapter will give you several ideas for finding new ways to add walking to your life.

The Family That Walks Together, Talks Together

In our rushed and hectic world, it's sometimes hard to find family "play time." You may be resisting a walking program because you don't want to take time away from your kids, spouse, or partner. You may feel that by walking every day, you'll cheat yourself out of important family time.

The solution? Get your family involved! Their support and encouragement will help keep you motivated when the going gets rough. And walking with your family gives you time to hear their concerns and problems. It also allows you be a role model for your kids. Wouldn't it be great if they began to value physical fitness early in life?

Take a look at this list of active family outing ideas. Add some you think your family would enjoy.

☐ Walk around a zoo or theme park.
☐ Discover local nature trails and hiking paths.
☐ Walk to the yogurt shop instead of driving.
☐ Take a picnic lunch and go for a walk at a local park.
☐ Walk with your kids to school.
☐ Encourage children to walk with their grandparents.
☐ _____
☐ _____
☐ _____

Hot Weather Hint: When exercising with children and older family members in hot, humid temperatures, remember that they are at greater risk for heat-related problems than you are. Make sure they get plenty of water before, during, and after exercise. Allow them to become accustomed to hot temperatures for a week to ten days before they exercise at a high intensity or for a long time.

Walking Makes Good Neighbors

What could be more convenient than a walking program that begins at your front door? Walking in the neighborhood is easy. And it's more fun if you have a neighbor or two who's willing to join you.

Chances are good that many of your neighbors also like to walk for exercise. When you're out walking, take a look at who is walking during that time of day. In no time at all, you'll be able to quickly spot the regulars. Then ask one or two if they'd like to join you.

Mall Walking: Shopping for an Indoor Walking Spot

If bad weather torpedoes your walking plans, you're not alone. But it doesn't have to be that way. Instead of quitting during bad weather, consider walking in a shopping mall. Malls are large, safe, well lighted, and climate controlled. They have wide, open walkways. Some people think that mall walking is boring. Not a chance! Malls are great for people-watching, and the scenery changes with each fashion season!

Many malls open their doors as early as six A.M. for walkers. Some even provide free coffee. The retail stores aren't open at that hour, so you won't have to dodge crowds and window shoppers. If you walk during store hours, however, you might be tempted to stray off course; if that's the case, leave your credit cards and cash at home.

Some malls encourage mall walking by sponsoring walking clubs and offering special events such as guest speakers and walk-a-thons. A mall in Dallas, Texas, lets walkers log into its "frequent shopper" computer when they walk during retail hours. Regular participation earns the walkers incentives such as discounts at mall stores.

And the mall is a great place to walk during the holidays. Think of it as a warmup for your shopping. It's possible that choosing the right gifts may even be easier because you will have gleaned lots of good ideas along the way. So instead of letting the hectic holidays put your walking program at risk, using shopping as an excuse to maintain and enhance your health and well-being.

Most communities have at least one mall. Contact the mall management office at the ones closest to your work (consider a lunch-time walk) and your home (for a walk before or after work). If the mall doesn't accommodate walkers, sell them on the idea! It's a great opportunity for malls to provide a community service, and retailers benefit from increased foot traffic.

Try Water Walking

Sometimes walking can be uncomfortable because of a painful sports injury, a chronic disease such as arthritis or osteoporosis, obesity, or other physical problems. If walking is painful for you, one solution is walking in water. Because your body is buoyant in water, it helps reduce the impact and pressure of weight-bearing activities on your bones and joints. This is an ideal solution for people who have joint problems or injuries.

Water also provides resistance, which causes you to work harder and burn a larger number of calories. If you've ever tried to walk in thigh- or chest-deep water, you know that it's difficult.

Finally, exercising in water is invigorating, relaxing, and fun, and water walking adds variety to your walking program.

WHERE TO FIND A POOL

Check out these sources of swimming pools that may be convenient to your home or work.

☐ YMCA or YWCA
☐ Schools and universities
☐ Swim and health clubs
☐ Park and recreation departments
☐ Hotel pools

At a public pool, you may also have access to a water aerobics class. This can introduce you to a variety of water exercises besides walking. A public pool also is more likely to have a lifeguard on duty—a necessary safety precaution if you're not an experienced swimmer.

If you have a backyard pool, walking in water is even more convenient. You don't need a standard lap pool at all. Small pools that are hip- to chest-deep are fine for water exercises.

If you've never learned to swim, take lessons. It's an important survival skill and allows you to enjoy recreational activities such as sailing, water skiing, snorkeling, and canoeing.

VARIATIONS OF WATER WALKING

Try the following activities in chest-deep water. Remember to warm up with a few stretches for at least 5 minutes before beginning, and cool down for another 5 minutes at the end of your session.

☐ Walk or skip forward and backward. Use the wall, a kickboard, or a rope for balance.
☐ Walk through the water moving your arms in a swim stroke motion.
☐ Alternate walking with swimming laps.
☐ Move your arms and legs as if you were skipping rope. Go backward and forward.

SAFETY TIPS
☐ Be aware of the water's depth and any potential hazards before getting in. Remember that swimming in open water, such as a lake or the ocean, has numerous risks including rocks, pollution, and currents.
☐ Never exercise in water alone, regardless of your skill level.
☐ Be courteous to others if you are sharing lanes in a lap pool.
☐ Know where the ladder and steps are located.

☐ Wear a waterproof stopwatch to monitor your time and heart rate.

☐ Wear waterproof sunscreen to protect against sunburn.

☐ Drink water frequently if you are exercising for a long period of time or if you're exercising vigorously. You can become dehydrated even while exercising in water.

Join a Walking Club—And Join the Crowd

Millions of people walk for exercise. And for companionship, many of them have joined together to form walking clubs. Walking clubs allow you to:

☐ meet new friends

☐ walk and talk with others

☐ participate in races

☐ learn new walking skills

To locate the walking clubs in your community, consult the weekend edition of your local paper for contact information. Or contact your city recreation department, the local YMCA, a health club, your walking shoe retailer, or any other sporting goods store. Some clubs request a nominal membership fee to cover the cost of newsletters and other educational information.

No walking clubs in your part of town? Then don't be shy—start one. Many newspapers offer free space for community groups to advertise their activities. The American Volksport Association can help you get a new walking club off the ground. Write or call them for more information (see page 137).

If walking near your workplace is easier, start a walking club in your company. Invite all of the employees to an organization meeting. If you find a lot of interest, you may want to have an early bird morning walking group, a lunch bunch, and an after-work wind-down group! Map out the routes and distances inside and outside of your building. During bad weather, encourage club members to walk at a shopping mall, if one is nearby. Once your walking club is established, conduct special promotions periodically to help retain members and recruit new ones.

Special Walking Events

Some organizations have events just for walkers. They are usually non-competitive outings open to people of all ages and physical abilities. Families and friends can stroll, walk, or jog. They can enjoy the scenery, stop for a picnic, and meet new friends along the way.

One example is volksmarching ("people walking"). Common in Europe, especially Germany, volksmarching was started to encourage families to walk together. The American Volksport Association (AVA) has more than 550 chapters nationwide which provide opportunities for walkers to join with others for fun and fitness. To get information about volksmarching events in your area, contact the national office (see page 137). As a member, you can receive a bi-monthly publication on volksmarching, plus lots of information on how to start a volksmarching club in your community.

Another European import is orienteering, a game that encourages walking. Orienteering participants use a map and a compass to navigate from one checkpoint to the next. Some participants compete for the best time; others simply enjoy being outdoors. Most enjoy the mental challenge of figuring out the best route for completing the course.

An orienteering course can be set anywhere, from the inner city to deep in a forest. Since these events bring together participants of all abilities, the courses at each meet are set at varying degrees of difficulty. Before each meet, an instructor teaches novice participants the necessary map reading and navigational skills.

If you like being outdoors and think you would enjoy being challenged mentally as well as physically, orienteering may be right up your alley. Check your local newspaper for information about clubs in your area or contact the U.S. Orienteering Federation (see page 137).

Take a Walking Vacation

What's *your* idea of a dream vacation? Lying in the sun on a white, sandy beach? Traveling cross-country in a camper? Taking a bus tour through Europe? While they sound relaxing, they definitely *won't* keep you in shape. In fact, people often report that vacations are one of the main reasons they fall off the walking wagon. When you're on vacation you're off your normal schedule and the routines of work and home, so activities like walking are often dropped.

Instead of thinking of a vacation as a chance to dump your walking program, think of it as a chance to boost your physical activity even more by walking everywhere. Walking is even better on vacation because it's a great way to see the sights, meet the natives, and have adventures that simply aren't available by bus or auto.

How To Take a Walking Vacation

Vacation	Ways to Walk
Beach resort	Kick up your heels on a sandy beach. Be sure to walk close to the water, where the sand is more compact; avoid walking long distances in loose, dry sand, which can strain the muscles in your calves and feet. Wear walking shoes if you walk for more than a few minutes. Watch out for dry sand in the heat of the day. It can be hot enough to burn the bottoms of your feet.
Cruise	Sign up with a cruise line that has ships with walking decks and exercise facilities. Many cruise lines have remodeled their ships to respond to the demands of health-conscious vacationers.
Golf	Walk the course instead of using a cart.
Car Trips	Plan stops each day to get out of the car and stretch your legs for a while. Or start each day with a hike or walking excursion to see the local sights before you move on.
Bus Tours	Make sure that the itinerary allows you free time to do what you want each day. Find out in advance where you can walk at each destination. Go with people who share your interest in walking. Consider taking a walking tour instead of an ordinary bus tour.
Camping	Make sure your camping destination has nature trails and hiking routes that you can access easily.
Family Reunions	Organize a family fun walk. Think of fun ways to make the walk interesting such as having each person "buddy up" with a first cousin. Have a walking version of a scavenger hunt.

If you're still at a loss as to how to plan a vacation that includes walking, get some help from a pro. Travel companies have sprung up all over the country to cater to the needs and interests of people who want active vacations. Such companies are listed in the classified section of most walking and fitness magazines. Or call your travel agent for information about walking vacations and other active getaways. Some companies have trips designed especially for singles, families, or other special interest groups.

Presidential Sports Award Program

The President's Council on Physical Fitness and Sports has a recognition and awards program designed to help people get physically fit and stay active. It's open to any person age 6 or older (participants between ages 6 and 13 must have their physical activity logs verified and signed by an adult). The council also has a Family Fitness Award for family members who participate in the program and earn awards together.

To qualify for the award, simply complete the requirements in one of sixty-seven physical activity categories within a four-month period. The three walking categories are Endurance Walking, Fitness Walking, and Race Walking. Just keep a log of your activities, and turn it in with a nominal handling fee to receive your award.

For more information contact Presidential Sports Award (see page 137).

Lend a Hand With Your Feet

Looking for fun? Try a walking special event. Almost anyone can join, and the camaraderie of joining others for fun, fitness, and philanthropy is hard to beat.

A good bet is your local American Heart Walk, sponsored by the American Heart Association. This is an annual walking event held in hundreds of communities around the country, usually in October. Corporate teams and individuals ask friends, family members, coworkers, clients, and vendors to sponsor their participation by making a tax-deductible donation.

The event promises a fun walk (distances vary by city), lots of great food, and a big dose of fresh air. Millions of dollars are raised yearly in hundreds of events nationwide. The AHA uses the proceeds from these events to support research to help fight heart disease and stroke. For more information about the American Heart Walk in your area, call your local American Heart Association at 1-800-242-8721. Other voluntary health agencies such as the American Cancer Society and the March of Dimes hold similar fund-raising events. You'll find that participating in a walking event can help your heart in more ways than one.

RUNNING/WALKING RACES

Road races have become popular Saturday morning events for many physically active people. Some sign up just to get in a good weekend workout. Others aim to reach a personal goal or set a personal record. Still others compete to win. An added bonus is that almost all of these races donate the proceeds to charitable organizations.

Most road races are either a "5K" or a "10K" (5 kilometers equals 3.1 miles, 10 kilometers equals 6.2 miles). Some races offer both categories. One-mile family fun runs are also popular. Runners and joggers predominate, but more and more exercise walkers participate each year.

Most walkers realize they're not going to win a prize for finishing first, second, or third—that's the runners' domain. Still, being outdoors and in a festive atmosphere is a healthy way to spend time with friends or family members. If it's tough to stay motivated to walk on the weekends, send in your entry fee for a weekend walking event. That's a good way to commit yourself to getting up and going on a Saturday morning.

If you plan to walk in a road race that includes runners, consider these tips:

☐ Start near the back of the pack. If you start too far to the front, you may get bumped and jostled by faster runners competing for good positions.
☐ Know your limitations. If you generally only walk a couple of miles a day, don't overextend yourself and sign up for a 10K.
☐ Don't be disappointed if you finish toward the end of the pack. Remember, you're just walking for fun. Many of the others are serious runners.

Walking Resources

Keep your walking program fresh and interesting by getting new ideas from walking groups and organizations. Here are a few that can help you with information about walking and about walking clubs and events. (Inclusion in this list does not constitute an endorsement, implied or otherwise, by the American Heart Association).

American Heart Walk
American Heart Association
National Center
7272 Greenville Avenue
Dallas, TX 75231
(800)242-8721

American Volksport Association
1001 Pat Booker Road, Suite 101
Universal City, TX 78148
(210)659-2112

Presidential Sports Award
P.O. Box 68207
Indianapolis, IN 46268-0207
(317)872-2900

Prevention Magazine Walking Club
33 E. Minor Street
Emmaus, PA 18098–0099
(610)967-5171

Rockport Walking Institute
220 Donald Lynch Boulevard
Marlboro, MA 01752
(508)485-2090

U.S. Orienteering Federation
P.O. Box 1444
Forest Park, GA 30051

Walking Magazine
Walking Inc.
9–11 Harcourt Street
Boston, MA 02116
(800)678-0881

Walking's Second Cousins

As regular walking becomes a habit, you may want to add new activities to spice up and vary your exercise program. The more physical activities you enjoy, the easier it will be to gain the fitness and health benefits you want from regular exercise. Plus, when you do a variety of activities, you work different muscle groups. This can help prevent overuse injuries. Certain activities, such as the ones described below, are logical and practical transitions from a regular walking program.

HIKING

Hitting the nature trail is a natural progression from fitness walking. Hiking takes your walking skills into a beautiful natural setting, over rough ground, and out in the elements. To do this successfully, you may need to change your footwear. For example, if the terrain is rough or rocky, the thin soles on your regular walking shoes won't protect your feet. Instead, you'll need a pair of rugged hiking boots with thick, hard rubber soles and ankle supports to prevent sprains.

Also, it's important to know your limits. You can't walk as fast over rough terrain, especially if it's uneven and uphill. Pace yourself, and don't overdo it. Be sure to watch where you're going. It's easy to get so caught up in the natural beauty that you don't realize how far you've walked, and getting back to the start may be difficult.

Be careful if your hike involves a big increase in altitude. You may need time to let your body adjust to the new altitude. You may need to walk more slowly and take more breaks. Always remember to drink plenty of water.

DANCING

When was the last time you spent an evening on the dance floor? Dancing is not only fun and exhilarating, it also exercises your heart and lungs.

Most types of dancing complement a walking program. For example, doing the waltz is about equal to brisk walking. Country and western dancing and line dancing have even more gusto, and will give you a good workout. So will disco and square dancing. Some people take ballet or tap dance lessons to help them keep in shape.

If you enjoyed dancing in the past, why not give it another whirl?

STAIR-CLIMBING

Want to beef up the intensity of your walking? It's simple—walk uphill. Of course, if you live in a place that doesn't have any hills, you'll find equal benefits in climbing stairs, and you'll find that stairs are everywhere. You can climb stairs during the day at the office, take the stairs instead of the elevator or escalator wherever you go, or work out on a stair-stepping machine at home or a local gym. Either way, keep the following precautions in mind.

☐ Be sure to warm up before you start climbing. Walking up stairs is a strenuous exercise, so be sure your body is ready for a vigorous workout.
☐ Wear comfortable shoes with a flat heel. Don't try to climb stairs in two-inch pumps. Your feet and calves will rebel!
☐ Know your limits. You may not be used to prolonged stair-

climbing. It's much harder than regular walking. So don't do too much at once.

☐ Place your whole foot, not just the ball of your foot, on each step. Otherwise, your calves are going to cave in and tighten up.

CROSS-COUNTRY SKIING

When you see a cross-country skier, the movements look effortless and beautiful. This popular winter sport is one of the best exercises around. Like walking, it requires significant effort on the part of your legs, back, arms, and abdominal muscles. Your arms move back and forth in a rhythmic fashion. The major difference between walking and cross-country skiing is that when you're walking, you use your arms mostly for balance, but with cross-country skiing, your arms work hard to propel you forward. As a result, cross-country skiing burns nearly twice as many calories as brisk walking.

Today, anyone can cross-country ski, whether or not there's snow on the ground. Dozens of exercise machines simulate the leg and arm actions of this vigorous activity. Try one at your local gym or YMCA.

If you're interested in buying a machine for your home, take our advice and try before you buy. Ask your exercise equipment dealer to let you try a skiing machine for at least a couple of weeks before investing money in one. You'll find that it requires a measure of balance and coordination—some people never seem to get the hang of it. If you're one of those, you'll regret buying something you'll never use. On the other hand, others get hooked on the ease and effectiveness of cross-country machines and they stay hooked—and fit—for life.

With walking, the good news is that life presents almost endless opportunities to get more exercise. Whether it's a shopping trip, a visit to the copier at work, or an outing to find a new place for lunch, almost anything can be turned into an opportunity to walk away with fun and fitness.

Appendix I
THE WALKING DIARY

Susan works as a manager for a large corporation. She and her husband Bill have two children, Eddie and Patty. Six months ago, when Susan's company started a wellness program for its employees, she decided that walking was the best way for her to participate and help keep her weight in check. She also thought walking was something she could do with her family and even her dog Rusty. This is Susan's sample diary for one week.

On the following pages, you'll find your own 12-week diary to fill in as you walk your way to a new, healthy, happy lifestyle. Good luck!

WEEK OF:

Goal(s): *To walk in my target heart zone at least 5 times this week for 25 minutes each time.*

_10/16_ to _10/22_ **Reward:** *Buy a new pair of walking shorts*

MONDAY

Where	Intensity	Time	Distance
Neighborhood	Heart rate = 127 (67% max. heart rate)	25 min.	1.4 mi.
work	RPE = 3	6 min.	?
	Daily Totals	31 min.	1.4 mi +

Comments: *Felt great to walk before work! It was so cool and refreshing. Raked leaves for half hour— a great workout for my arms!*

TUESDAY

Where	Intensity	Time	Distance
Neighborhood	Heart rate = 115 (66% max. heart rate)	30 min.	1.7 mi.
work	RPE = 3	18 min.	1 mi.
	Daily Totals	48 min.	2.8 mi.

Comments: *Bill walked with me this morning—what fun! And I almost doubled my daily goal! So glad I had my walking shoes in the car so I could walk with my co-workers.*

WEDNESDAY

Where	Intensity	Time	Distance
To and from library	easy	20 min.	.5 mi.
Highland Park	Heart rate = 120 (67% max. heart rate)	25 min.	1.4 mi.
Neighborhood	RPE = 2	5 min.	?
	Daily Totals	50 min.	1.9 mi.

Comments: *Missed my walk this morning but made up for it by walking around the bleachers at Eddie's soccer game! I'm proud of my creativity!*

THURSDAY

Where	Intensity	Time	Distance
Shopping mall	RPE = 3	15 min.	.75 mi.
	Daily Totals	15 min.	.75 mi.

Comments: *A crazy day! Missed my walk, but at least I managed something. It poured for most of the day— I need a light rain suit.*

*Rate your intensity by using one of the following methods. List whether your walk was easy, moderate, or hard. You can also use a rating of perceived exertion (RPE), a percent of maximum heart rate, or state whether or not you stayed in your target heart rate zone. See pages 44–45 for more information on measuring walking intensity.

FRIDAY

Where	Intensity	Time	Distance
Neighborhood	Heart rate = 127 (70% max. heart rate)	30 min.	1.8 mi.
work	RPE = 3	6 min.	?
	Daily Totals	36 min.	1.8 mi +

Comments: _Spent 45 minutes on the dance floor with Bill. What a romantic way to stay in shape! What a difference a day makes._

SATURDAY

Where	Intensity	Time	Distance
Wildlife Preserve	RPE = 3–6 (going up hills)	85 min.	4.7 mi.
	Daily Totals	85 min.	4.7 mi.!

Comments: _The most I ever walked, with beautiful things to see every step of the way. I'd forgotten how much I love nature!_

SUNDAY

Where	Intensity	Time	Distance
To church	easy	10 min.	.5 mi.
	Daily Totals	10 min.	.5 mi.
	Weekly Totals	275 min.	13.8 mi.

Comments: _A day of rest, but walking to church did help me limber up._

WEEKLY SUMMARY

Attained Weekly Goals?
☑ Yes. My reward is _new shorts._
☐ No, but close
☐ No, pretty far off, but I'll try again next week

Did Daily Essentials?
☑ Warm-up
☑ Cool-down
☑ Stretches

Comments: _Good week! Nearly lapsed when it rained on Thursday but doing something felt better. Can't believe I walked 13 miles in a week! Haven't lost weight but I feel wonderful!_

Other Activities (list what, where, with whom, amount):
Raked leaves; dancing with Bill; cleaned garage; 20 curl-ups and 15 modified push-ups 3 times this week.

Goal(s) for next week:
To walk in my target heart rate zone for 30 minutes on at least 4 days, plus a 60-minute walk or hike on Saturday.

WEEK OF: Goal(s): _____

_____ to _____   Reward: _____

MONDAY

Where	Intensity	Time	Distance
	Daily Totals		

Comments: _____
_____
_____

TUESDAY

Where	Intensity	Time	Distance
	Daily Totals		

Comments: _____
_____
_____

WEDNESDAY

Where	Intensity	Time	Distance
	Daily Totals		

Comments: _____
_____
_____

THURSDAY

Where	Intensity	Time	Distance
	Daily Totals		

Comments: _____
_____
_____

144

FRIDAY

Where	Intensity	Time	Distance
	Daily Totals		

Comments: _____
_____
_____

SATURDAY

Where	Intensity	Time	Distance
	Daily Totals		

Comments: _____
_____
_____

SUNDAY

Where	Intensity	Time	Distance
	Daily Totals		
	Weekly Totals		

Comments: _____
_____

WEEKLY SUMMARY

Attained Weekly Goals?
☐ Yes. My reward is _____
☐ No, but close
☐ No, pretty far off, but I'll try again next week

Did Daily Essentials
☐ Warm-up
☐ Cool-down
☐ Stretches

Comments: _____
_____
_____

Other Activities (list what, where, with whom, amount):
_____
_____

Goal(s) for next week:
_____
_____

WEEK OF:

_____ to _____

Goal(s): _____

_____

Reward: _____

MONDAY

Where	Intensity	Time	Distance
	Daily Totals		

Comments: _____

_____

TUESDAY

Where	Intensity	Time	Distance
	Daily Totals		

Comments: _____

_____

WEDNESDAY

Where	Intensity	Time	Distance
	Daily Totals		

Comments: _____

_____

THURSDAY

Where	Intensity	Time	Distance
	Daily Totals		

Comments: _____

_____

FRIDAY

Where	Intensity	Time	Distance
	Daily Totals		

Comments: _____
_____
_____

SATURDAY

Where	Intensity	Time	Distance
	Daily Totals		

Comments: _____
_____
_____

SUNDAY

Where	Intensity	Time	Distance
	Daily Totals		
	Weekly Totals		

Comments: _____
_____
_____

WEEKLY SUMMARY

Attained Weekly Goals?
☐ Yes. My reward is _____
☐ No, but close
☐ No, pretty far off, but I'll try again next week

Did Daily Essentials
☐ Warm-up
☐ Cool-down
☐ Stretches

Comments: _____
_____
_____

Other Activities (list what, where, with whom, amount):
_____
_____

Goal(s) for next week:
_____
_____

WEEK OF: _____   Goal(s): _____

_____ to _____   Reward: _____

MONDAY

Where	Intensity	Time	Distance
	Daily Totals		

Comments: _____

_____

_____

TUESDAY

Where	Intensity	Time	Distance
	Daily Totals		

Comments: _____

_____

_____

WEDNESDAY

Where	Intensity	Time	Distance
	Daily Totals		

Comments: _____

_____

_____

THURSDAY

Where	Intensity	Time	Distance
	Daily Totals		

Comments: _____

_____

_____

FRIDAY

Where	Intensity	Time	Distance
	Daily Totals		

Comments: _____
_____
_____

SATURDAY

Where	Intensity	Time	Distance
	Daily Totals		

Comments: _____
_____
_____

SUNDAY

Where	Intensity	Time	Distance
	Daily Totals		
	Weekly Totals		

Comments: _____
_____

WEEKLY SUMMARY

Attained Weekly Goals?　　　　　　　　　Did Daily Essentials
☐ Yes. My reward is _____　☐ Warm-up
☐ No, but close　　　　　　　　　　　☐ Cool-down
☐ No, pretty far off, but I'll try again next week　☐ Stretches

Comments: _____
_____
_____

Other Activities (list what, where, with whom, amount):
_____
_____

Goal(s) for next week:
_____
_____

WEEK OF: Goal(s): _____

_____ to _____   Reward: _____

MONDAY

Where	Intensity	Time	Distance
	Daily Totals		

Comments: _____

_____

_____

TUESDAY

Where	Intensity	Time	Distance
	Daily Totals		

Comments: _____

_____

_____

WEDNESDAY

Where	Intensity	Time	Distance
	Daily Totals		

Comments: _____

_____

_____

THURSDAY

Where	Intensity	Time	Distance
	Daily Totals		

Comments: _____

_____

_____

FRIDAY

Where	Intensity	Time	Distance
	Daily Totals		

Comments: _____
_____
_____

SATURDAY

Where	Intensity	Time	Distance
	Daily Totals		

Comments: _____
_____
_____

SUNDAY

Where	Intensity	Time	Distance
	Daily Totals		
	Weekly Totals		

Comments: _____
_____

WEEKLY SUMMARY

Attained Weekly Goals?
☐ Yes. My reward is _____
☐ No, but close
☐ No, pretty far off, but I'll try again next week

Did Daily Essentials
☐ Warm-up
☐ Cool-down
☐ Stretches

Comments: _____
_____
_____

Other Activities (list what, where, with whom, amount):
_____
_____

Goal(s) for next week:
_____
_____

WEEK OF:

_____ to _____

Goal(s): _____

Reward: _____

MONDAY

Where	Intensity	Time	Distance
	Daily Totals		

Comments: _____
_____
_____

TUESDAY

Where	Intensity	Time	Distance
	Daily Totals		

Comments: _____
_____
_____

WEDNESDAY

Where	Intensity	Time	Distance
	Daily Totals		

Comments: _____
_____
_____

THURSDAY

Where	Intensity	Time	Distance
	Daily Totals		

Comments: _____
_____
_____

FRIDAY

Where	Intensity	Time	Distance
	Daily Totals		

Comments: _____
_____
_____

SATURDAY

Where	Intensity	Time	Distance
	Daily Totals		

Comments: _____
_____
_____

SUNDAY

Where	Intensity	Time	Distance
	Daily Totals		
	Weekly Totals		

Comments: _____
_____

WEEKLY SUMMARY

Attained Weekly Goals?
☐ Yes. My reward is _____
☐ No, but close
☐ No, pretty far off, but I'll try again next week

Did Daily Essentials
☐ Warm-up
☐ Cool-down
☐ Stretches

Comments: _____
_____
_____

Other Activities (list what, where, with whom, amount):
_____
_____

Goal(s) for next week:
_____
_____

153

WEEK OF: Goal(s): _____

_____ to _____ Reward: _____

MONDAY

Where	Intensity	Time	Distance
	Daily Totals		

Comments: _____

_____

_____

TUESDAY

Where	Intensity	Time	Distance
	Daily Totals		

Comments: _____

_____

_____

WEDNESDAY

Where	Intensity	Time	Distance
	Daily Totals		

Comments: _____

_____

_____

THURSDAY

Where	Intensity	Time	Distance
	Daily Totals		

Comments: _____

_____

_____

Where	Intensity	Time	Distance
	Daily Totals		

Comments: _____
_____
_____

SATURDAY

Where	Intensity	Time	Distance
	Daily Totals		

Comments: _____
_____
_____

SUNDAY

Where	Intensity	Time	Distance
	Daily Totals		
	Weekly Totals		

Comments: _____
_____

WEEKLY SUMMARY

Attained Weekly Goals?
☐ Yes. My reward is _____
☐ No, but close
☐ No, pretty far off, but I'll try again next week

Did Daily Essentials
☐ Warm-up
☐ Cool-down
☐ Stretches

Comments: _____
_____
_____

Other Activities (list what, where, with whom, amount):
_____
_____

Goal(s) for next week:
_____
_____

WEEK OF: Goal(s): _____

_____ to _____ Reward: _____

MONDAY

Where	Intensity	Time	Distance
	Daily Totals		

Comments: _____
_____
_____

TUESDAY

Where	Intensity	Time	Distance
	Daily Totals		

Comments: _____
_____
_____

WEDNESDAY

Where	Intensity	Time	Distance
	Daily Totals		

Comments: _____
_____
_____

THURSDAY

Where	Intensity	Time	Distance
	Daily Totals		

Comments: _____
_____
_____

FRIDAY

Where	Intensity	Time	Distance
	Daily Totals		

Comments: _____
_____
_____

SATURDAY

Where	Intensity	Time	Distance
	Daily Totals		

Comments: _____
_____
_____

SUNDAY

Where	Intensity	Time	Distance
	Daily Totals		
	Weekly Totals		

Comments: _____
_____

WEEKLY SUMMARY

Attained Weekly Goals?
☐ Yes. My reward is _____
☐ No, but close
☐ No, pretty far off, but I'll try again next week

Did Daily Essentials
☐ Warm-up
☐ Cool-down
☐ Stretches

Comments: _____
_____
_____

Other Activities (list what, where, with whom, amount):
_____
_____

Goal(s) for next week:
_____
_____
_____

WEEK OF: Goal(s): _____

_____ to _____   Reward: _____

MONDAY

Where	Intensity	Time	Distance
	Daily Totals		

Comments: _____
_____
_____

TUESDAY

Where	Intensity	Time	Distance
	Daily Totals		

Comments: _____
_____
_____

WEDNESDAY

Where	Intensity	Time	Distance
	Daily Totals		

Comments: _____
_____
_____

THURSDAY

Where	Intensity	Time	Distance
	Daily Totals		

Comments: _____
_____
_____

FRIDAY

Where	Intensity	Time	Distance
	Daily Totals		

Comments: _____
_____
_____

SATURDAY

Where	Intensity	Time	Distance
	Daily Totals		

Comments: _____
_____
_____

SUNDAY

Where	Intensity	Time	Distance
	Daily Totals		
	Weekly Totals		

Comments: _____
_____
_____

WEEKLY SUMMARY

Attained Weekly Goals?
☐ Yes. My reward is _____
☐ No, but close
☐ No, pretty far off, but I'll try again next week

Did Daily Essentials
☐ Warm-up
☐ Cool-down
☐ Stretches

Comments: _____
_____
_____

Other Activities (list what, where, with whom, amount):
_____
_____

Goal(s) for next week:
_____
_____

WEEK OF:

Goal(s): _____

_____ to _____

Reward: _____

MONDAY

Where	Intensity	Time	Distance
	Daily Totals		

Comments: _____
_____
_____
_____

TUESDAY

Where	Intensity	Time	Distance
	Daily Totals		

Comments: _____
_____
_____
_____

WEDNESDAY

Where	Intensity	Time	Distance
	Daily Totals		

Comments: _____
_____
_____
_____

THURSDAY

Where	Intensity	Time	Distance
	Daily Totals		

Comments: _____
_____
_____

FRIDAY

Where	Intensity	Time	Distance
	Daily Totals		

Comments: _____
_____
_____

SATURDAY

Where	Intensity	Time	Distance
	Daily Totals		

Comments: _____
_____
_____

SUNDAY

Where	Intensity	Time	Distance
	Daily Totals		
	Weekly Totals		

Comments: _____
_____

WEEKLY SUMMARY

Attained Weekly Goals?
☐ Yes. My reward is _____
☐ No, but close
☐ No, pretty far off, but I'll try again next week

Did Daily Essentials
☐ Warm-up
☐ Cool-down
☐ Stretches

Comments: _____
_____
_____

Other Activities (list what, where, with whom, amount):
_____
_____

Goal(s) for next week:
_____
_____

WEEK OF: Goal(s): _____

_____ to _____   Reward: _____

MONDAY

Where	Intensity	Time	Distance
	Daily Totals		

Comments: _____

TUESDAY

Where	Intensity	Time	Distance
	Daily Totals		

Comments: _____

WEDNESDAY

Where	Intensity	Time	Distance
	Daily Totals		

Comments: _____

THURSDAY

Where	Intensity	Time	Distance
	Daily Totals		

Comments: _____

FRIDAY

Where	Intensity	Time	Distance
	Daily Totals		

Comments: _____

_____

_____

SATURDAY

Where	Intensity	Time	Distance
	Daily Totals		

Comments: _____

_____

_____

SUNDAY

Where	Intensity	Time	Distance
	Daily Totals		
	Weekly Totals		

Comments: _____

_____

WEEKLY SUMMARY

Attained Weekly Goals?   Did Daily Essentials
☐ Yes. My reward is _____   ☐ Warm-up
☐ No, but close   ☐ Cool-down
☐ No, pretty far off, but I'll try again next week   ☐ Stretches

Comments: _____

_____

_____

Other Activities (list what, where, with whom, amount):

_____

_____

Goal(s) for next week:

_____

_____

WEEK OF: _____ Goal(s): _____

_____ to _____ Reward: _____

MONDAY

Where	Intensity	Time	Distance
	Daily Totals		

Comments: _____

_____

_____

TUESDAY

Where	Intensity	Time	Distance
	Daily Totals		

Comments: _____

_____

_____

WEDNESDAY

Where	Intensity	Time	Distance
	Daily Totals		

Comments: _____

_____

_____

THURSDAY

Where	Intensity	Time	Distance
	Daily Totals		

Comments: _____

_____

_____

FRIDAY

Where	Intensity	Time	Distance
	Daily Totals		

Comments: _____
_____
_____

SATURDAY

Where	Intensity	Time	Distance
	Daily Totals		

Comments: _____
_____
_____

SUNDAY

Where	Intensity	Time	Distance
	Daily Totals		
	Weekly Totals		

Comments: _____
_____

WEEKLY SUMMARY

Attained Weekly Goals?
☐ Yes. My reward is _____
☐ No, but close
☐ No, pretty far off, but I'll try again next week

Did Daily Essentials
☐ Warm-up
☐ Cool-down
☐ Stretches

Comments: _____
_____
_____

Other Activities (list what, where, with whom, amount):
_____
_____

Goal(s) for next week:
_____
_____

WEEK OF:

Goal(s): _____

_____

_____ to _____ Reward: _____

MONDAY

Where	Intensity	Time	Distance
	Daily Totals		

Comments: _____
_____
_____

TUESDAY

Where	Intensity	Time	Distance
	Daily Totals		

Comments: _____
_____
_____

WEDNESDAY

Where	Intensity	Time	Distance
	Daily Totals		

Comments: _____
_____
_____

THURSDAY

Where	Intensity	Time	Distance
	Daily Totals		

Comments: _____
_____
_____

FRIDAY

Where	Intensity	Time	Distance
	Daily Totals		

Comments: _____
_____
_____

SATURDAY

Where	Intensity	Time	Distance
	Daily Totals		

Comments: _____
_____
_____

SUNDAY

Where	Intensity	Time	Distance
	Daily Totals		
	Weekly Totals		

Comments: _____
_____

WEEKLY SUMMARY

Attained Weekly Goals?
☐ Yes. My reward is _____
☐ No, but close
☐ No, pretty far off, but I'll try again next week

Did Daily Essentials
☐ Warm-up
☐ Cool-down
☐ Stretches

Comments: _____
_____
_____

Other Activities (list what, where, with whom, amount):
_____
_____

Goal(s) for next week:
_____
_____

Appendix II
SCORING THE ONE-MILE FITNESS TEST

Age	Heart Rate	Men		Women	
		A	B	A	B
20–29	110	19:36	17:06	20:57	19:08
	120	19:10	16:36	20:27	18:38
	130	18:35	16:06	20:00	18:12
	140	18:06	15:36	19:30	17:42
	150	17:36	15:10	19:00	17:12
	160	17:09	14:42	18:30	16:42
	170	16:39	14:12	18:00	16:12
30–39	110	18:21	15:54	19:46	17:52
	120	17:52	15:24	19:18	17:24
	130	17:22	14:54	18:48	16:54
	140	16:54	14:30	18:18	16:24
	150	16:26	14:00	17:48	15:54
	160	15:58	13:30	17:18	15:24
	170	15:28	13:01	16:54	14:55
40–49	110	18:05	15:38	19:15	17:20
	120	17:36	15:09	18:45	16:50
	130	17:07	14:41	18:18	16:24
	140	16:38	14:12	17:48	15:54
	150	16:09	13:42	17:18	15:24
	160	15:42	13:15	16:48	14:54
	170	15:12	12:45	16:18	14:25
50–59	110	17:49	15:22	18:40	17:04
	120	17:20	14:53	18:12	16:36
	130	16:51	14:24	17:42	16:06
	140	16:22	13:51	17:18	15:36
	150	15:53	13:26	16:48	15:06
	160	15:26	12:59	16:18	14:36
	170	14:56	12:30	15:48	14:06
60+	110	17:55	15:33	18:00	16:36
	120	17:24	15:04	17:30	16:06
	130	16:57	14:36	17:01	15:37
	140	16:28	14:07	16:31	15:09
	150	15:59	13:39	16:02	14:39
	160	15:30	13:10	15:32	14:12
	170	15:04	12:42	15:04	13:42

Credits: Adapted with permission from *Living With Exercise*, by Steven N. Blair, P.E.D., Director of Epidemiology at the Cooper Institute for Aerobics Research in Dallas, American Health Publishing Company, 1991, 1-800-736-7323). All rights reserved. The One-Mile Fitness Test is based on maximal oxygen uptake estimates from studies done by Dr. James M. Rippe and colleagues. *JAMA* 1988; volume 259:2720–2724.

Appendix III
PERSONAL DATA RECORD

| Interval | One-Mile Fitness Test | | | | Body Weight | Blood Pressure | Blood Cholesterol | Other |
	Date	Time	Heart Rate	Fitness Category				
Baseline								
One Month								
Two Months								
Three Months								
Six Months								
Nine Months								
One Year								

Appendix IV
WALKING MILESTONES

Date	Milestone Description

Appendix V
AMERICAN HEART ASSOCIATION AFFILIATES

American Heart Association
National Center
Dallas, Texas

AHA, Alabama Affiliate, Inc.
Birmingham, Alabama

AHA, Alaska Affiliate, Inc.
Anchorage, Alaska

AHA, Arizona Affiliate, Inc.
Tempe, Arizona

AHA, Arkansas Affiliate, Inc.
Little Rock, Arkansas

AHA, California Affiliate, Inc.
Burlingame, California

AHA of Metropolitan Chicago, Inc.
Chicago, Illinois

AHA of Colorado/Wyoming Inc.
Denver, Colorado

AHA, Connecticut Affiliate, Inc.
Wallingford, Connecticut

AHA, Dakota Affiliate, Inc.
Jamestown, North Dakota

AHA, Delaware Affiliate, Inc.
Newark, Delaware

AHA, Florida Affiliate, Inc.
St. Petersburg, Florida

AHA, Georgia Affiliate, Inc.
Marietta, Georgia

AHA, Hawaii Affiliate, Inc.
Honolulu, Hawaii

AHA of Idaho/Montana
Boise, Idaho

AHA, Illinois Affiliate, Inc.
Springfield, Illinois

AHA, Indiana Affiliate, Inc.
Indianapolis, Indiana

AHA, Iowa Affiliate, Inc.
Des Moines, Iowa

AHA, Kansas Affiliate, Inc.
Topeka, Kansas

AHA, Kentucky Affiliate, Inc.
Louisville, Kentucky

AHA, Greater Los Angeles Affiliate, Inc.
Los Angeles, California

AHA, Louisiana Affiliate, Inc.
Destrehan, Louisiana

AHA, Maine Affiliate, Inc.
Augusta, Maine

AHA, Maryland Affiliate, Inc.
Baltimore, Maryland

AHA, Massachusetts Affiliate, Inc.
Framingham, Massachusetts

AHA of Michigan, Inc.
Lathrup Village, Michigan

AHA, Minnesota Affiliate, Inc.
Minneapolis, Minnesota

AHA, Mississippi Affiliate, Inc.
Jackson, Mississippi

AHA, Missouri Affiliate, Inc.
St. Louis, Missouri

AHA, Nation's Capital Affiliate, Inc.
Washington, D.C.

AHA, Nebraska Affiliate, Inc.
Omaha, Nebraska

AHA, Nevada Affiliate, Inc.
Las Vegas, Nevada

AHA, New Hampshire Affiliate, Inc.
Manchester, New Hampshire

AHA, New Jersey Affiliate, Inc.
North Brunswick, New Jersey

AHA, New Mexico Affiliate, Inc.
Albuquerque, New Mexico

AHA, New York City Affiliate, Inc.
New York, New York

AHA, New York State Affiliate, Inc.
North Syracuse, New York

AHA, North Carolina Affiliate, Inc.
Chapel Hill, North Carolina

AHA, Northeast Ohio Affiliate, Inc.
Cleveland, Ohio

AHA, Ohio Affiliate, Inc.
Columbus, Ohio

AHA, Oklahoma Affiliate, Inc.
Oklahoma City, Oklahoma

AHA, Oregon Affiliate, Inc.
Portland, Oregon

AHA, Pennsylvania Affiliate, Inc.
Camp Hill, Pennsylvania

Puerto Rico Heart Association, Inc.
Hato Rey, Puerto Rico

AHA, Rhode Island Affiliate, Inc.
Pawtucket, Rhode Island

AHA, South Carolina Affiliate, Inc.
Columbia, South Carolina

AHA, Southeastern Pennsylvania Affiliate, Inc.
Conshohocken, Pennsylvania

AHA, Tennessee Affiliate, Inc.
Nashville, Tennessee

AHA, Texas Affiliate, Inc.
Austin, Texas

AHA, Utah Affiliate, Inc.
Salt Lake City, Utah

AHA, Vermont Affiliate, Inc.
Williston, Vermont

AHA, Virginia Affiliate, Inc.
Glen Allen, Virginia

AHA, Washington Affiliate, Inc.
Seattle, Washington

AHA, West Virginia Affiliate, Inc.
Charleston, West Virginia

AHA, Wisconsin Affiliate, Inc.
Milwaukee, Wisconsin

INDEX

∽

Acetaminophen, 118
Achilles tendonitis, 121
Activity barriers, identifying, 2–4
Advanced walking, 35, 97
   hand weights in, 97–98
   race walking in, 100
   resistive cords in, 99–100
   stair-climbing machines in, 101
   treadmills in, 100–101
   walking/jogging in, 100
   walking poles in, 99
Aerobic exercise, 5–6
   adding to fitness routine, 103
   benefits of, 5–6
   lifetime benefits from, 106–7
   low-intensity, 7–8
   moderate, 7
   various types of, 6–7
Air pollution, and walking, 82
Alternate thigh stretches, 78
American Cancer Society, 136
American Heart Association
   affiliates of, 175–76
   recommendations on aerobic activity, 6
   recommendations on fat consumption, 112, 114
   walking guidelines for heart patients, 124
American Heart Walk, 135, 137
American Volksport Association (AVA), 132, 133, 137
Anti-inflammatories, 118
Aquatic stretches and calisthenics, 131–32

Arthritis, 130
Aspirin, 118

Balanced Fitness Assessment, 108–9
Bicycling, 9
   calories burned in, 13
Binge eating, 115
Blisters, 120
   prevention of, 63
Blood pressure, reducing, 6
Breathing, 75–76
Bursitis, 121

Calcium, 113
Calf stretches, 70, 79
Calisthenics, 104
Calories
   burning, in workout, 13, 116
   and weight control, 115
Carbohydrates, 111–12
Cardiovascular exercise equipment, 100–101
   costs involved in, 10–11
Cardiovascular fitness, 5–6
Cartilage tears, 121
Chest pull, 69
Chest stretch, 68
Chondromalacia, 121
Clothes
   impact of weather on, 82–85
   for walking, 63
Cold, exercising with common, 118–19
Cold weather, walking in, 82–83
Complex carbohydrates, 111–12

Compression in treating walking injuries, 118

Cool-downs
in strength-building program, 106
stretches for, 77–79

Cooper Institute for Aerobics Research, vii

Corns, 120

Cross-country skiing, 139

Dairy products, 113–14

Dancing, 138

Darkness, walking in, 81

Dehydration, 84

Diabetes, 3, 6

Diet. *See* Nutrition

Dogs, and safe walking, 81

Elevation in treating walking injuries, 118

Exercise(s)
aerobic, 5–7, 103, 106–7
for better posture, 73–74
dislike for, 3
reasons for, 1–2
strength training, 5

Exercise approach to walking, 36–37

Exercise-related injury
risk of, 79–80
strength-building in preventing, 105

Exercising, excuses for not, 2–4

Family outings, 128–29

Fasting, 115

Fats, 112–13

Fitness level, determining, 30–32

Fitness program, balancing your, 102–9

Fitness walking, 34–35

F.I.T.T. formula, 36–37

Flexibility, 102

Frostbite, 82–83

Fun, walking for, 3, 16–17, 95–96

Goal Ladder, 55–56

Goals, setting, 21, 49–56

Gymnastics, 5

Hamstring stretches, 70

Hand weights, 97–98
methods for using, 98
safety tips for, 98

High-density lipoprotein (HDL) cholesterol, 6, 17

Health problems, walking for, 3–4

Healthy Heart Food Pyramid, 110–11

Heart, benefits of walking to, 5–6, 8, 10, 18, 124

Heart attack
contributing factors for, 124
controllable risk factors for, 124
risk of, during exercise, 4
warning signs for, 80

Heart disease risk factors
fat consumption as, 112
walking in modifying, 17, 18

Heart patients, walking for, 124–26

Heart rate, target, 42–44

Heat exhaustion, 84

Heatstroke, 84

Heel bruise, 120

Heel counter, 58

Heel spur, 120

High altitude, and walking, 82

High blood pressure, reducing, 3, 6

Hiking, 137–38

Hot weather, walking in, 84–85, 129

Hydration tips, 64–65

Hypothermia, 82–83

Ibuprofin, 118

Ice in treating walking injuries, 117

Injuries, preventing, 79–80, 105

Inner thigh stretch, 78

Jogging, 5, 9, 10, 100
calories burned in, 13

Jumping jacks, 132

Kickboard press, 131

Lacing techniques for walking shoes, 61–62

Lapse, preventing, 23, 92–95

Low-density lipoprotein (LDL) cholesterol levels, 113

Leg lifts, 132

Lifestyle approach to walking, 37–38
  advantages and disadvantages to, 39–40
  clothes for, 63–64
  Talk Test for pacing, 41, 77
  time spent walking in, 45
  use of pedometer in, 90–91
  warming up in, 71
Lifestyle changes
  making stick, 25–28
  need for medical ok, 28–30
Locations, suggested, for walking, 11–12
Low-back pain, relief from, 73, 75
Low-intensity activities, 7–8

Mall walking, 129–30
March of Dimes, 136
Massage, 107–8
Medical okay, need for, 28–30, 124–25
Milk, fat content of, 113–14
Moderate exercise, 7
Monounsaturated fats, 113
Morton's Neuroma, 120
Motivation, 20, 86–96
Mountain sickness, symptoms of, 82
Muscle symmetry, improving, 105
Muscular strength, 103–4

Neck stretches, 67
Nutrition
  carbohydrates in, 111–12
  dairy products in, 113–14
  fats in, 112–13
  proteins in, 114
  serving sizes in, 112
  taking good, in stride, 110–11

Obesity, and walking, 127
Older walkers, 3
  tips for, 126–27
One-mile walking test, 32–33
  preparing for, 30
  scoring, 31–32, 169
Orienteering, 133
Osteoporosis, 6, 104, 130
Outdoors, walking, 80–81
Overload, 105
Overuse injuries, preventing, 105

Pace, determining, for walking, 76–77
Pedometers, 90–91
Perceived exertion, 41
Perceived Exertion Scale, 41–42
Personal Data Record, 32, 86–87, 171
Personal safety, and walking, 81–82
Physical activity, types of, 5
Plantar fasciitis, 120
Polyunsaturated fats, 113
Positive thoughts, power of, 23–24
Posture
  exercises for, 73–74
  importance of, 71–74
  proper standing, 72, 73
Power walking, 97
Pregnancy, walking in, 122–23
Presidential Sports Award, 137
Presidential Sports Award Program, 135
President's Council on Physical Fitness and Sports, 135
Prevention Magazine Walking Club, 137
Progression, 105
Protein, 114
Purposeful walking, 34

Race walking, 100
Racquet sports, 10
Rain, walking in, 83–84
Rating of Perceived Exertion (RPE), 41–42
Reflective clothing, and walking, 81
Rep, 106
Resistance, adding, in advanced walking, 99–100
Resistive cords, 99–100
Rest in treating walking injuries, 117
Rewards from walking, 22, 91–92
R-I-C-E principles, 117–18
Risks, unwillingness to take, 54
Road races, 136
Rockport Walking Institute, 137
Running, 10
  calories burned in, 13
Running/walking races, 136

Saturated fat, 113
Sesamoiditis, 120
Set, 106
Shoes. *See* Walking shoes

Shoulder circles, 68
Side bends, 69
Simple carbohydrate, 112
Sit-ups, 131
Skiing, 9
    cross-country, 139
Smoking, walking in breaking habit of,
        76
Social life, and walking, 18–19
Socks, 62–63
Specificity, 106
Sports drinks, 65
Stair-climbing, 10, 138–39
Stair-climbing machines, 101
Stone bruise, 120
Strength building
    benefits of, 105
    activities for, 103, 104
Strength training
    cool-downs in, 106
    exercises in, 5
    rules in, 105–6
    warm-ups in, 106
Stress management, 17–18
Stretching
    activities, 5
    aquatic, 131–32
    cool-down, 77–79
    exercises for, 66–71
    importance of, 66, 79
Stroke
    contributing factors for, 124
    controllable risk factors for, 124
Sunscreen, 64
Swayback, 73
Swimming, 5, 9
    calories burned in, 13

Talk Test
    in gauging workout intensity, 41, 45,
        76
    as ideal for lifestyle-oriented walking,
        41, 77
Target heart rate, 42–44
    determining, with coronary artery dis-
        ease, 125
    table for, 44
Tendonitis, 121
Thigh stretches, 78

Traffic, and walking, 81
Treadmills, 100–101
Triggers, controlling, 21–22

U.S. Orienteering Federation, 133, 137
Unsaturated fats, 113

Volksmarching, 133

Walking, 5, 17
    advanced, 35, 97–101
    avoiding injuries in, 4, 79–80, 105
    barriers to, 53–54
    benefits of, 8, 9–18
    breathing in, 75–76
    calorie burning in, 13, 116
    as challenge to heart, 10
    changing behavior in, 22–23
    clothes for, 63–64
    controlling triggers in, 21–22
    cool-down stretches for, 77–79
    costs involved in, 3, 10–11
    determining proper pace for, 76–77
    finding locations for, 11–12
    finding opportunities for, 128–39
    fitness, 34–35
    frequency for, 40–41
    for fun 3, 16–17, 95–96
    for heart patients, 124–26
    importance of posture for, 71–74
    importance of stretching for, 66, 79
    intermixing with jogging, 100
    involving friends in, 22
    lapses in, 23, 92–95
    long-term benefits from, 18–20
    and low-back pain, 75
    as low risk, 12
    measuring stride in, 90–91
    motivation for, 20
    need for water during, 64–65, 85
    obesity, 127
    outdoors, 80–81
    pacing in, 41–44
    power of positive thinking in, 23–24
    purposeful, 34
    race, 100
    reasons for, 14–16
    reasons for making lifetime habit, ix–
        x

recording progress in, 20–21
related activities, 137–39
resources for, 136–37
rewards in, 22, 91–92
safety in, 81–82
setting goals in, 21, 49–56
short-term benefits from, 17–18
skill level for, 14
special events in, 133, 135
staying motivated in, 86–96
and stress management, 17–18
strolling in, 13
style of, 79
surface for, 79
time factor in, 13, 45
timing length of, 89–91
tips for older walkers, 126–27
types of, 33–35
warm-ups for, 66–71
water, 130–31
and weight control, 114–16
Walking clubs, 35, 81, 132
Walking diary, 21, 87–89, 141–68
Walking events, special, 133, 135
Walking gait, basic elements of good,
    74–75
Walking injuries
pain relief for, 118
preventing, 117
R-I-C-E formula for, 117–18
treating specific, 120–21
Walking/jogging, 100

Walking magazine, 137
"Walking Milestone" record, 91, 173
Walking plan
choosing right, 36–40
customized, 46–48
Walking poles, 99
Walking shoes, 3, 11
checklist for buying, 60
deciding to buy, 59–61
finding right, 57–59
lacing techniques, 61
need for new, 61–62
as safety factor, 79
Walking vacation, 133–35
Warm-ups, 66–71, 107–8
benefits of, 66
in strength-building program, 106
stretching exercises in, 66–71
Water, need for, while walking, 64–65,
    85
Water walking, 130–31
Water safety, 131
Weather, impact of clothing on, 82–85
Weight-bearing exercise, 10
Weight control, 18
role of walking in, 114–16
Weightlifting, 5, 10, 102, 104
Workout
calories burned in 30-minute, 13
evaluating rate of, 77
Workout intensity table, 45

Yoga, 5, 102